THE
WEIGHT LOSS
HYPNOSIS SOLUTION

By Joshua Seth, Cht

The Weight Loss Hypnosis Solution:
How To Lose Weight Permanently
Without Diets or Willpower

Copyright © 2008 by Joshua Seth, CHt

ISBN 978-0-9818472-0-7
Library of Congress Control Number 2008908899

Published By:

New You Publishing
3867 W. Market t. Suite 123
Fairlawn, OH 44333
http://www.weightlosshypnosissolution.com

Disclaimer: Every effort has been made to accurately represent our program and it's potential. Any claims made of actual weight loss or examples of actual results can be verified upon request. The testimonials, examples, and claims used are exceptional results, don't apply to the average purchaser and are not intended to represent or guarantee that anyone will achieve the same or similar results. Each individual's success depends on his or her background, dedication, desire and motivation. As with any self improvement endeavor, there is an inherent risk of loss of time and capital and there is no guarantee that you will lose weight. Please consult your doctor before starting any weight loss program. All information contained within these pages is the opinion of the author and is not intended as medical advice. This product is not intended to diagnose, treat, cure, or prevent any disease.

The author of this book is not a medical doctor. Doing anything recommended or suggested in this book must be done at your own risk. The author and publisher specifically disclaim any liability resulting from the use or application of the information contained in this book. This disclaimer is included because of the increasingly litigious nature of our society and the widespread misinformation about both weight loss and hypnosis.

v 1.2

To Habibtee

TABLE OF CONTENTS

To claim your free gifts (valued at $97) visit www.joshuaseth.com/bonus

Real People. Real Results.

Lost 17 Pounds In 5 Weeks

"Dear Joshua, I attended your hypnosis session on the Caribbean Princess on Feb. 9. It was the last full day of the cruise and like most everyone else, I over-indulged (food-wise) the whole cruise. But attending your session got me started on a weight loss program. As of today (April 18th), I have lost 17 lbs. I feel so much better! My clothes fit better and physically I have more energy. I want to thank you for your motivational talk, that really got me moving"

Thanks again,

Joseph So
Toronto, Canada

Gave Up Soft Drinks With No Caffeine Headaches

"I sat through your seminar for weight loss on Sat afternoon. Was very intrigued as I knew I needed to "give up" the diet Coke. I had my last "drink" of the stuff on Sun a.m., actually throwing the entire can away and have not wanted one since and it has been 6 weeks now. In fact the thought of having a diet Coke is just repulsive."

Sharon Hoover
Oklahoma City, OK

PS - I don't know if it was the hypnosis or not, but I did not have any headaches from the lack of caffeine.

Amazing!

"I am finding myself eating much, much slower, moving my food around on my plate, not eating another bite until the one in my mouth is totally chewed!!!! Amazing."

Vilinda Lemons
Bryan, OH

I've Taken Charge Of My Life

"First, I thought it was impossible for me to be influenced by hypnosis. Wrong, I was and as such, since that very day, I've stayed the course and revised my eating habits without variance. In addition, I combined (the hypnosis sessions) with 1/2 hr per day of walking in the pool. Weight loss is slow but steady. Combined with exercise, I feel more enthusiastic about living each day. As a stroke survivor nearly 1 year ago, combined with diabetes, I've taken charge of my life and live each day to it's fullest. I do like the idea of finally fitting into my clothes without bulges."

Irv Roth
Boynton Beach, Florida

Lost 14 Pounds In 25 Days

"I attended your weight-loss seminar on a cruise. I noticed at my next meal I didn't eat all the food on my plate. Then I started using the smaller plates and still not eating it all. In our cabin I listened to your CD's that I'd bought. I started eating even less. I have listened to the CD's every day since we got home. It has been 25 days and I have already lost 14 pounds! I feel great and know that this will continue to work! Thanks, Joshua"

Sue Chantry
Ogden Utah

To claim your free gifts (valued at $97) visit www.joshuaseth.com/bonus

The Weight Is Slowly But Effectively Coming Off

"I Have tried lots of diets to lose the 20+ pounds that keep returning and I was tired of always feeling guilty about everything I ate. I had resigned myself to be the size I was. Then on the cruise I attended your hypnosis show and sat in the back ready to leave.

But I started to feel like I was being hypnotized when I was watching the people on stage. I was impressed with the show since it was highly entertaining and not demeaning to the participants. When you offered the weight loss seminar I figured I may as well see what you had to say.

In that session I was hypnotized and told things I had heard a zillion times about weight loss but the whole attitude about the positive outlook and 'the feel good' and 'I can do it now' that was the emphasis I really heard.

It worked. Without consciously thinking about it that evening I had taken slow small bites, put my fork down, thought about the food and the taste and actually left some food on my plate because I felt full. Seems simple enough but I had not been brought up that way. I even refused dessert for the first time on a cruise since nothing seemed appealing enough.

It actually wasn't until the next day that I realized I was doing the food control without a guilt trip or serious mind games in order to decide whether to eat something or not. It was just happening! I could hardly wait to get home and do my 21 days with the CD. It worked. I really do look forward to the sessions and I lost the first 5 lbs over Christmas. I feel better and now people are starting to notice the difference. I am so glad I went to your show and thanks again ofr all the support as I work through my 6 CD Weight Loss program. I feel no pressure doing the program and the weight is slowly but effectively coming off!"

Diane Meacher
North Vancouver, BC

Lost Over 12 Pounds

"I bought your weight loss program on my last cruise, after hearing your seminar. I thought you might like to know what's been going on for me since then.

I have managed to lose 12 1/2 pounds more since coming home. [Since I am only 5 feet tall, a total of 12 1/2 pounds makes a considerable difference]. I look at sugary desserts now as something I don't want; so it is much easier to resist them. I find myself listening to my body more. When I have an impulse to eat something, I start for the refrigerator; and when I reaize I'm not really hungry, I close the fridge door without taking anything. It feels good to be in control.

Thank-you, thank-you, thank-you for sharing your sensible and positive approach to weight loss. I found it resonated with me and has been very helpful.

Sincerely, Davida Schachter,
Lakewood, N.J.

Easily Stopped Drinking Sodas And Eating Cookies

"Hi Joshua,

I ordered your weight-loss CDs about a week and a half ago. I can't believe how easy it's been for me to stop drinking sodas and eating cookies!! I'm sure anyone who reads this will think I'm paid to post stuff like this but I'm not- just a real person who is REALLY digging your CD's!

I've lost 4 pounds already :-) But more importantly, I am definitely feeling better about myself and I feel happier already.

I was thin/average for my entire life until two years ago when I gained 20 lbs. During my conscious programming (which I definitely think has helped me "reinforce" while I'm at work!) I even figured out the emotional trigger that caused my weight gain.

I just wanted to say a big THANK YOU!! If 4 lbs is all I lose I'll still be happy! I feel great about myself, and have found that your CD's relieve a great deal of my stress too!

Joshua, BIG HUG!!"

Sherri Buete
Palmetto, Florida

To claim your free gifts (valued at $97) visit www.joshuaseth.com/bonus

My Doctor Is Thrilled

"I am having wonderful success with the weight loss cd. I have been using it in conjuction with weight watchers point system. The combination in awesome and a great deal of fun. Lossing slowly but surely my Doctor is thrilled and of course so am I."

Alice Arfa
Hallandale, FL

Chocolate Cravings Disappeared

"Cruise ships are designed to make you gain weight. I attended Joshua's hypnosis session on overeating just before the Norwegian Dream invited passengers to their chocoholic buffet. I couldn't believe that I was then able to walk through the buffet and only take pictures — and I love chocolate. I'm a believer!"

Carole Goodfellow
Livonia, Michigan

Become All You Are Created To Become

"Joshua… I saw your great stage show and attended your weight loss seminar. It's great to know you have dedicated your life to help others bring out their potential. I'm a big believer in God and draw much strength from Him or Her…but also believe God uses people like yourself to discover and become all we were created to become. Thanks again for a great seminar and for being a positive force in this world."

Dave Schnider
Kitchener, Ontario

73 Years Old And Lost 17 ½ Pounds

"Joshua, Let me share my story with you, since you have made such a difference.

I am 73 and have the typical problems of a male my age:

Enlarging prostate, high blood pressure, and a borderline diabetic.

That of course means I have an enlarged belly and nothing I have tried in the past years has made a difference. Until your weight loss session and CD.

I was in your afternoon session on a cruise in mid-September.

I was convinced I could not be hypnotized. But, I gave it a try.

I lost about 15 minutes of my life that afternoon and "woke" very refreshed. And, I waited in line to buy your CD.

We were traveling for another 2 weeks, so I was unable to listen to your CD until October 1. That was the first time I was conscious enough to here the suggestions you were planting.

I became a believer and faithfully for 22 days, I listened to the CDs.

Life interrupted, and I thought I would re-start your program one day. But, to my surprise, the pounds seemed to drop.

I consciously ate less, concentrated on what I ate, and stopped snacking.

Today, the day after Thanksgiving, I found I have lost 17 ½ pounds. I actually lost weight on Thanksgiving.

I do not feel deprived of food. If I want a sweet treat, I have it.

But those are becoming further apart.

Thank you for the difference you have made in my life."

Dr. Charles Frank
Waxhaw, NC

To claim your free gifts (valued at $97) visit www.joshuaseth.com/bonus

67 Years Old And Lost 19 Pounds!

"Hi Joshua,

I attended your seminar last Nov/Dec on a cruise ship and bought your tape. I am 67 and have had a weight problem for the past several years. I also have MS and do not get as much exercise as I should. However I happily noticed my weight go down as my portion control set in. I have lost 19 lbs. and it continues slowly but steadily. I also found another side effect from the tape. Last week I hurt my shoulder and was in a great deal of pain so that it awakened me during the night with movement. After listening to my tape and going through the relaxation part the next morning the pain was almost gone. By the next morning after listening to the tape I truly felt so good! Thank you for enhancing my life."

Shirley DeNeire
Atlantis, Florida

Stopped Feeling Guilty

"I recently returned from a 17 day cruise. Imagine all that good food, relaxing and having a good time, but for me a constant worry is weight gain while on holidays, from over eating and lack of exercise (I lost approx 60 lbs about 4 years ago and it is a constant stuggle to maintain that loss).

It was during this cruise that I had the opportunity to meet Joshua. In fact I ended up being part of his evenings' show. I was so impressed with Joshua that I went to his weight loss seminar a few days later. I attribute the fact that I attended this seminar as the reason I had very little weight gain. After the seminar it didn't seem to matter that I didn't fill my plate up with unnecessay food and that I didn't feel guilty with leaving food on my plate. Yes, I did eat differently than I would had I been home but, I ate normal portions and I certainly didn't overindulge like I would have in the past. So, thank you Joshua and keep on helping people."

Wendy Fort
Logan Lake, BC

To claim your free gifts (valued at $97) visit www.joshuaseth.com/bonus

Lost 10 Pounds in 6 Weeks

"Joshua: By listening to your tape regularly…and doing "mindful eating"…(as of May 16th) I've lost 10 lbs. since returning from the cruise on April 28th. Keep up the good work. You have my vote… your method is preferable over pills, potions and whatnot."

Edward A. Solustri
Orange Park, Florida

Lost 20 Pounds

"Just this January I purchased your Total Weight Loss System and for the first time I stuck with it and had lost around 15 pounds when I fell and broke my leg. Without really thinking about it, I have stayed with the changes I made using your system thru this difficult time and I have lost an additional 5 pounds."

Janice Pelton
Niwot, Colorado

Feels Better About Herself

"Thank you so much for the weight loss hypnosis CD. I listen to it every day it helps me with many areas of my life. For one thing I no longer eat any food in front of the T.V.! I had a bad habit of getting popcorn and eating to much of it mindlessly in front of the T.V. Now I sit at the table for all my meals, even snacks. The foods that I eat now are healthy. It is fantastic that you helped me to feel better about myself. My goals are definitley reachable with your help."

Cherie Regueiro
Akron, Ohio

A Remarkable Experience

"I had remarkable experiences with Joshua Seth's Weight Loss CD. I was on the Coral Princess in December 2007 and saw him at one of the shows. My son's name is Seth Joshua and I felt a draw to see Joshua Seth. I was a participant on the stage and truly was hypnotized. After the show; I purchased the CD on Weight Loss and a couple of other CDs that he was selling. The Weight Loss CD has really helped me and I have learned to take control of my weight gain. Thank you so much."

Loryn Halperin
Parkland, Florida

Feels More Positive and Confident

"I already feel more positive and confident that I CAN do this! I am not interested in the food as much!!! WOW!!!! THANKS SO MUCH! I am "in" for this amazing journey and believe I can do it with your support! Again, thanks for the great program! I am feeling a positive difference each day!"

Fran Anderson
Ontario, Canada

Lost 15 Pounds And Proved Her Mother In Law Wrong

"I was on a Princess cruise on January 2008. You had a hypnosis session. I went to it along with my mother-n-law. She said that it would probably never work. Well you helped me prove to her that it does work. I have lost a total of 15 pounds.

And I feel great thanks to you."

Bobbi Belasco
Barnegat, NJ

To claim your free gifts (valued at $97) visit www.joshuaseth.com/bonus

Lost 13 Pounds In 7 Weeks

"I purchased one of Joshua's Hypnosis for Weight Loss CD's while on a Cruise in January 2007. When I returned home I promptly put it with the rest of the junk I had accumulated on the cruise and forgot about it.

After battling with my weight for years, I finally joined a gym in March 2008 but was still over eating. Then I remembered Joshua's CD and decided "what the heck, I couldn't hurt to try it". Sometime during the 21 days I listened to the CD I started noticing that the way I looked at food had changed. I no longer wanted the chocolate bars and cookies every night after dinner. Instead I have fruit or nuts when I need a snack and that isn't often now. I've also changed the way I cook, adding more vegetables and less meat and starch. I feel better and have lost 13 pounds in seven weeks. The program really works! Thank you Joshua."

Stacey Gordon
Montara, Calif.

Lost 7 Pounds In 3 Weeks

"I recently completed your 21 day Weight Loss CD session and have lost 7 pounds (approx. 3% of my previous weight) during that time.

I have found that not only have I lost the weight but my eating habits have changed for the better! I am eating more reasonable portions of food for meals and have stopped "grazing" between meals. Needless to say I am totally satisfied with the results of your weight loss program.

I have found that unlike other weight loss programs I have tried, this one not only results in weight loss, but has an unexpected benefit as well: I experience calm and tranquility while listening to the CDs. I find myself looking forward to the sessions and have no problem working them into my daily schedule. Thanks."

John Shenal
Chesterfield, Virginia

To claim your free gifts (valued at $97) visit www.joshuaseth.com/bonus

Took In A Notch On The Belt

"I think the enjoy every bite (suggestion on the CD) is helping me slow down my intake. I am retired military, and have always gulped my food fast. I have taken in one notch on the belt. Even my skeptical wife can notice the change and my sister in law here in Germany can't understand why I am not eating much."

Milton Fritts
Germany

A True Breakthrough

"Hello Joshua,

My husband and I were on the Coral Princess Panama Canal cruise and he was hypnotized by you on stage the first show. Then we attended the group session on board for "those of us wanting to lose weight and gain control". Because we were impressed, we bought the CD's and have enjoyed them so much.

I want you to know that the Confidence Session has been a true breakthrough for me and even tho' I have passed my 21 days (on day 29) I still listen every day to be immersed in your soothing voice and to treat myself to the relaxation and support it gives me. I use my anchor prn (retired nurse) and feel myself being more self-assured "in every way"! I'm now using the Lose Weight CDs as well. ;>)

Best wishes to you and thank you for my new-found state of confidence!"

Emily Shenal
Chesterfield, Virginia

ABOUT THIS BOOK

I developed this program in the middle of the ocean far from the sight of land but within easy reach of an endless buffet. Yes, I created the techniques detailed within these pages aboard a cruise ship. Actually, aboard dozens of cruise ships. You see, for over two years I travelled the world aboard some of the largest and most extravagant cruise ship vessels ever created. Once a week I would perform my stage hypnosis show in a beautiful 1,000 seat showroom for the passengers on that voyage, and then I would become one of those passengers myself, enjoying all the many ports of call throughout the world and feasting on the round-the-clock parade of food that is the buffet. Endless mountains of cookies and cakes piled high amidst the glistening arraignments of pastries and pies. Never ending, always changing, and available twenty-four hours a day, seven days a week to delight my taste buds and while away the many leisurely hours of my endless summer. Ahhh, what a life.

After the first few months of this routine I noticed that I was having trouble closing the clasp on my suit pants. Most of the week was spent lounging about in shorts and a t-shirt, but on that one night a week when I performed my stage act it was becoming harder and harder to fit into my suit. My girlfriend Suzy noticed the same thing. She's a dancer and usually stick thin, but now she had developed this plump little pouch for the first time in her life. So we rode the elevator up to the gym on the 16th floor and weighted ourselves.

It shouldn't have been such a shock to find that I had gained over 10 pounds, but believe me, it was. I had been the same weight since college and now I was fat. Not obese, but still, fat. Not good for an entertainer. Certainly not good for a hypnotist. Most people are aware that hypnosis is one of the most effective methods for losing weight ever created. I knew this. I'd studied this. Heck, I'm a certified hypnotherapist through the National Guild of Hypnotists and had helped many people with this issue in the past. But now I had become the one who needed help.

There's nothing quite so motivating for losing weight as having your super hot girlfriend slowly rub your big belly with a sad look on her face and say "What happened to my Habibee?" (she's from Lebanon, and Habibee is Arabic for "my love") That was it. It was time to review all the weight loss material I had studied over the years and apply it to myself. When we hit the next port of call in an English speaking country I didn't head for the beach, instead I took a cab straight to a supersized bookstore and loaded up on all the weight loss reference materials I could find. I tore apart everything I thought I knew about this issue and rebuilt it from the ground up. I threw out everything that was based in the big lie of the diet industry (explained in Chapter 4) and simplified everything that worked, using myself as the guinea pig.

I started using the techniques found within these pages on myself and within a few short weeks had lost those extra pounds and returned to my original weight. I've stayed there ever since, but more importantly, I now have more energy than ever before and feel better in every way. Over the next couple of years of touring the world on cruise ships, I still had access to all the same foods but I never gained any more weight. I began desiring fruit instead of frosting, carrots instead of cookies. I didn't even have to choose between them because I'd successfully reprogrammed my subconscious mind to desire healthy foods. My inner mind was doing all the work for me and all I had to do was act on it.

To claim your free gifts (valued at $97) visit www.joshuaseth.com/bonus

By using the power of my own mind to control my food cravings and eliminate overeating, I was able to solve a problem in my own life that has become a huge issue for over a third of the population in the US. Over one hundred twenty million Americans are now considered obese according to their body mass index (BMI). This represents a 61% increase since 1991 and the trend is continuing to worsen. Obesity causes over 300,000 deaths a year and is quickly becoming an epidemic in the United States.

I believe that the main reason we are each put on this Earth is to become the best example of a person we can be while helping other people become the best they can be along the way. This is the reason I've written this book. If these techniques can work for me while surrounded by an endless parade of food on a cruise ship they can work for you too.

This isn't just idle boasting. Soon after I developed *The Weight Loss Hypnosis Solution* I started conducting seminars on the topic every week on the cruises. Now, after conducting over 100 of these seminars, tens of thousands of people have been able to lose weight and keep it off using this method. You've already read some of their stories in the first few pages of this book. They are truly inspiring. They come from different backgrounds, in different places, and are of vastly different ages, but what they all share in common is that they made a decision to change their lives using *The Weight Loss Hypnosis Solution* and are now living examples of what is possible when you apply these techniques to yourself.

It has been my privilege to help so many people along the way and it is my sincere wish that you will soon become one of these success stories yourself. You are not alone on this journey. I offer you continued support and dialogue through my blog at www.JoshuaSeth.com. I am committed to helping you reach your goals, transform your life, and live your dreams. This book is the first step.

The journey will change your life.

Joshua Seth, CHt

To claim your free gifts (valued at $97) visit www.joshuaseth.com/bonus

YOUR $97 BONUS GIFT!

I'd like to give you a generous helping of weight loss Articles, MP3s, and Videos worth $97 absolutely free. Why am I doing this? Because I want you to become a part of my growing online community, full of people just like you who are committed to improving their lives. I regularly publish new articles designed to help you live the life of your dreams, but I can't help you if I don't know how to reach you. So I'm piling on the bonuses here as a way to get you to join my list and keep this process going week after week.

When you sign up at www.joshuaseth.com/bonus I'll instantly send you $97 worth of bonus materials you can put to use immediately. I'll also email you my weekly newsletter at no charge. If you ever get tired of hearing from me (which I hope never happens) a simple click on the Unsubscribe link at the bottom of any of my emails will take you off the list. What I'm really looking for though is a way to help you reach your goals on an ongoing basis.

Commitment to losing weight is important (you've demonstrated your commitment by buying and reading this book) but it's not enough. You must also have consistency. Commitment to losing weight today plus consistency of action tomorrow is what will create the results you're looking for. That's why I want to keep sending you motivational emails, to keep you on track each and every week.

To claim your free gifts (valued at $97) visit www.joshuaseth.com/bonus

The book you hold in your hands is part of a larger system designed to help you lose weight, without diets or willpower, and keep it off permanently. The written word is somewhat limiting when dealing with this topic. Some materials lend themselves better to audio (the Hypnosis CDs) and some to video (the Emotional Freedom Technique). The online articles will update and expand upon the ideas explored within these pages. Taken together these resources comprise a complete weight loss solution designed to help you reach your ideal weight as quickly and easily as possible.

As a purchaser of this book, I would like to give you additional resources that would never fit between it's covers. These free bonus gifts are ready and waiting for you now. To claim them, simply visit...

www.joshuaseth.com/bonus

CHAPTER I
What's Eating You?

If you are overweight, and you are like most people, you may have already spent hundreds of dollars on unused gym memberships, have an attic filled with useless cooking gadgets, and a garage cluttered with expensive exercise equipment that only gave you temporary results at best.

Have you spent hundreds or possibly thousands of dollars on special weight loss foods, shakes, and diet pills? Have you gone to doctor after doctor, asking for a miracle pill, or diet, or fad exercise, that would make you skinny?

Do you have a closet full of fat clothes, skinny clothes and clothes for when you're in between?

Do you have old skinny you pictures hanging in your home to remind you of 'the way we were' because you looked so good, and now you're feeling a bit queasy to see your current, perhaps a bit overweight self pictured around your home?

Have you reached the point yet of avoiding full-length mirrors, even if you have to turn sideways (and that doesn't help either) to avoid seeing what you look like in reality? Do you avoid looking at cars for fear you'll see a reflection of your butt in the windows as it goes by?

To claim your free gifts (valued at $97) visit www.joshuaseth.com/bonus

Have you reached a point where you will not let your spouse or significant other see the light reflect off your nude body anymore? Are you afraid to see yourself in a bikini? Do you want the light turned off before you start making love? Are you getting a little paranoid about your body?

Have you decided that it's time for you to lock yourself away in your home on weekends due to your embarrassment over being heavy? Has your weight problem drained you of all self-confidence and affected your work?

How about your energy levels? Have they dipped down to the point of exhaustion since you've put on those extra pounds? Has it gotten harder for you to get up off that couch and do what needs to be done?

Maybe you are blaming your weight issue on other problems in your life. Or perhaps it's the other way around and you are blaming your lack of progress in your career on your weight. Whatever the reason you give yourself, the time has come to make a change. You are ready for it now or you wouldn't have picked up this book.

This book was written because there are millions of people who have gone through what you are experiencing. Millions of people are searching for a natural, drug free, permanent weight loss solution. You are not alone.

Simple Math

Losing weight is a very basic equation: You must burn more calories than you consume. Every pound you gain represents 3500 calories you didn't need to eat.

Every pound you lose represents 3500 calories that you burned off that you normally don't.

We each burn a certain number of calories per day for our normal and automatic bodily functions. The burning of calories represents energy conversion for the operation of our body. In technical terms, energy to fuel our physical plant.

Our simple body functions, such as breathing and digestion, burn calories so that the entire organism, the body that everyone sees and loves, works properly.

Depending on your height, weight and metabolism, the amount of calories that you burn daily will vary. There are some medical conditions that can slow down your metabolism and those certainly need to be addressed by your doctor.

Losing weight translates to knowing and remembering one simple fact: to lose weight you must burn more calories than you consume. That's the formula. It's easy to say but hard to do, right?

Now, let's get started with giving you a solution that will help you to achieve permanent weight loss. I'm gonna get you motivated to lose weight, to set goals for yourself and reach them, and to address all the other issues that have stopped you from losing weight in the past. You will succeed this time, and more easily than you ever thought possible.

This program is unique because it incorporates tools that address your own individual needs and works with your own self defined goals. Everyone has unique physical differences, emotional differences, psychological differences and body types after all.

We also have different mindsets regarding food, exercise, and body image. This system will help you custom-tailor your own program to fit your lifestyle, your schedule, and most importantly, your own individual needs. It will help you create the body you want so you can live a life you'll love.

To claim your free gifts (valued at $97) send a blank email to bonus@joshuaseth.com

All of us live different lives and have different lifestyles. You might be a stay-at-home parent, a single parent, living in a home where both you and your spouse are a working couple, or perhaps you're single without kids.

No matter whether you are the CEO of a Fortune 500 corporation or you are in middle management, this program will work for you. Perhaps you are an Administrator or an Assistant; it will work for you too. It doesn't matter if you work outdoors, or indoors, no matter what your life dictates or directs - you are going to design this program to work for you without turning your life upside down. This program is a true weight loss solution. It has worked for thousands of people just like you.

Your habits are going to change while you easily and effortlessly lose weight. The major thing that you need to remember is that YOU are responsible for making this happen. Only you can change your life. You can't do it for anyone else. You do it for yourself because you deserve to be healthy, fit, vibrant, and full of life.

In this program there are no special foods to purchase. There are no pills to take, no drops to put on your tongue, no scented aromatherapy oils to put on your mind's eye either.

You don't have to eat an excessive amount of any food. You are not denied any foods, nor are you required to starve yourself ever.

Yes, this system is designed to fit into your busy day. You'll never have to give up one moment of your social activities to go to a group meeting.

And you can eat, whenever you want, not at a fixed time like many programs demand.

Most importantly, this system will help you take control of your weight and your life permanently.

From this moment on, you'll no longer be a slave to negative thoughts or food obsessions. You will be empowered to become who you really are inside, beautiful, perfect, and free.

Using this system, you'll lose the weight you want, feel better about yourself, and once and for all succeed.

The Obesity Epidemic

The obesity epidemic has become a major issue over the past 20 years, even while more and more time and money is being spent trying to solve it.

In 1990, the total number of overweight adults in the United States was approximately 58 million. By the year 2000 it had already ballooned to over 100 million. Today 120 million Americans are not only overweight, but obese (according to the Center for Disease Control's own statistics).

From 1960 to 2002, the average weight jumped from:

• Men: 166.3 pounds to 191 pounds

• Women: 140.2 pounds to 164.3 pounds

• Body mass index for adults (ages 20-74) has increased from 25 to 28

Today, the Most Recent Statistics from the CDC (The Center for Disease Control) Indicate that:

• Two-thirds of adults in the U.S. are overweight or obese.

• As many as 30 percent of U.S. children are overweight.

• Childhood obesity has more than doubled within the past 25 years.

If you are a part of this statistic, or know someone who is, you should be aware that having a serious weight issue can put you at risk for:

- Diabetes

- Heart Disease

- Stroke

- Hypertension

- Gallbladder Disease

- Sleep Apnea

- Osteoarthritis

- Certain forms of Cancer

Being obese can contribute to:

- High cholesterol

- Menstrual irregularities

- Pregnancy complications

- Hirsutism (facial hair growth)

- Depression

The heath risks of carrying extra weight are enormous. Excess weight can literally become a life or death issue if it's not managed correctly.

- Percentage of cardiovascular disease cases related to obesity: Nearly 70 percent

- Effect of obesity on blood pressure: More than doubles one's chances of developing high blood pressure

It's important to be responsible for your own eating habits. At the end of the day you are the only one who is.

It's time for you to honestly fill out the assessment forms on the following pages. They will help you better understand where you are now and where you want to go from here. This is an important step. Don't skip it. Grab a pen and fill in these assessment forms before we continue. You'll be glad you did.

YOUR EMOTIONAL EATING HABITS

I eat when I am feeling:

Anxious:	____ Yes	____ No
Afraid:	____ Yes	____ No
Bored:	____ Yes	____ No
Frustrated:	____ Yes	____ No
Happy:	____ Yes	____ No
Hungry:	____ Yes	____ No
Hyperactive:	____ Yes	____ No
Lonely:	____ Yes	____ No
Nervous:	____ Yes	____ No
Stressed:	____ Yes	____ No
Sad:	____ Yes	____ No

WHERE DO YOU EAT?

I snack or overeat when I'm:

At Parties:	____ Yes	____ No
Sporting Events:	____ Yes	____ No
On Coffee Breaks:	____ Yes	____ No
In Bed:	____ Yes	____ No
In The Car:	____ Yes	____ No
When Reading:	____ Yes	____ No
While Watching TV:	____ Yes	____ No

To claim your free gifts (valued at $97) send a blank email to bonus@joshuaseth.com

DO YOU REWARD YOURSELF WITH FOOD?

I reward myself with food whenever I need:

Attention: ____Yes ____No

A Distraction: ____Yes ____No

Comfort: ____Yes ____No

Companionship: ____Yes ____No

Love: ____Yes ____No

Something To Do: ____Yes ____No

To Change My Mood: ____Yes ____No

To Feel Important: ____Yes ____No

To Feel Secure: ____Yes ____No

To Relax: ____Yes ____No

Sex: ____Yes ____No

YOUR IDEAL WEIGHT

Start With The End In Mind:

1. Why do you want your weight to change?

   _____

   _____

2. What do you want your weight to be?

   _____

   _____

3. Why did you chose this particular weight?

   And what would your ideal weight be if we threw out those reasons?

   _____

   _____

4. What age were you the last time you weighed that amount?

   _____

   _____

5. Recognizing that you are older now and that change is a part of life, is your answer to question #2 above appropriate and attainable?

   If it is, then that number represents your ideal weight.

My Ideal Weight Is: _____

YOUR FUEL GAUGE

For the first three weeks of this program you should eat whenever you are hungry and your hunger level is in the 1-2 range on the following gauge. This may mean eating meals at unusual times of the day, or possibly even more often.

Stop eating when you reach the Third Quarter. To determine where you are on the fuel gauge, whenever you are about to eat, place your hand on your stomach as a way of directing attention to that area of the body. Close your eyes and concentrate on your hunger level. Reconnect your mind with your body so you can feel what you need to do. Don't rely on outside influences (like parties or certain times of day). Rely on yourself.

Use the following gauge to judge your hunger level. Eat slowly, chew your food, be mindful of what you are eating, and from time to time place your hand on your stomach to reassess your level of hunger.

Level E (Empty)

Your stomach is uncomfortably empty. You are starving. *It is important to eat before you get to this level.* (Your metabolism slows down so your body will be more efficient at storing fat for the coming famine.)

First Quarter

You cannot feel the presence of food in your system from the previous meal and you are hungry. (This is the point at which you should start eating.)

Second Quarter

This is how you feel when you've just eaten and are comfortably digesting the food. (You do not feel any hunger at these levels.)

Half Full

You are eating and beginning to feel satisfied.

Third Quarter

You are comfortable and satisfied. *You don't feel hungry or uncomfortable from overeating.* (This is when you should stop eating.)

Fourth Quarter

You have gone beyond the level of comfort by either eating too much or too fast (or both). *After eating you feel uncomfortable, heavy, dull, and listless.*

Full

You can't eat another bite. Your stomach is full and feels like it's going to burst.

Eat until you feel satisfied - not until you feel full.

To claim your free gifts (valued at $97) send a blank email to bonus@joshuaseth.com

CHAPTER 2
Why Have You Decided To Lose Weight Now?

Introspection is a great way to begin your journey to becoming the new you. Look inside to discover why you want to change, and want to change now. This can have a tremendous impact on your success.

Have you considered the reasons why you've made the decision to lose weight now? What's your motivation? Is it to get into that bathing suit for the summer, a dress for a friend's party, or general health and wellness?

Do you realize today how much better you felt when you carried a few pounds less? Do you want to have more energy and be more active instead of listlessly dragging your belly around? Do you have a nagging health issue that only serious and permanent weight loss would make more manageable for you? Do you want to feel better about yourself? List the top three reasons you want to start losing weight today.

I want to lose weight starting right now because:

1. _____

2. _____

3. _____

The 4 Types Of Overweight People

There are 4 major categories of people who are overweight. Read each of these descriptions to determine in which group you belong. You may belong to one specific group or a combination of groups:

1. Medical conditions and/or medications. Many medical conditions require medications, cause inflammation, retention of water, and weight gain. This can make it hard to take off the weight. Before beginning any program, you should consult with your physician.

2. Lack of motivation to exercise and eat properly. Sometimes people call this "being lazy", although that's really not a fair description. It really comes down to a lack of belief in your own ability to successfully become the person you'd like to be. When you have a clear mental and emotional connection to your outcome, the motivation to achieve it becomes automatic. Until that happens though, you're likely to remain a typical couch potato.

3. Cravings and attraction to fatty or sugary foods. Let's face it almost everyone craves a sloppy cheeseburger and fries or a piece of chocolate cake every now and then. That's OK! It's even OK to eat it once in a great while. It's when this type of eating becomes your daily routine that it gets dangerous to your waistline, not to mention your heart, your arteries, your blood pressure, and your overall health and well being.

4. Emotional/Self-Esteem Issues. Think about this for a moment: When you're upset, hurt, or angry do you head for the refrigerator or the pantry? Are your emotions attached to food? Do you reward yourself with food? Does food make you feel better about yourself, even if only temporarily? If you answered "yes" to any of those questions, you could have an emotional attachment to food.

Review all four categories and determine which ones apply to you.

This process is not complicated, but it may require looking at these issues from a new angle. Instead of focusing on food and keeping yourself from it we are going to focus on the positive: becoming the person you truly want to be. Traditional weight loss solutions focus on the negative (ie deprivation) and that is why they so rarely achieve the desired results.

Let's explore the two most common methods for weight loss, willpower and diets, and discover why they don't work for most people. Then I'll reveal how using your mind to change your body is a much easier and far more effective way to achieve your goals.

CHAPTER 3
Why Willpower Won't Work

When conducting weight loss seminars as I do around the country, I always start by asking the following question, "By a show of hands, who here has attempted, in the past, to use will power to lose weight?" And then hundreds of hands go up simultaneously, almost everybody in the room.

This scenario is very common. Most people try using willpower to lose weight first. Willpower, as you probably know, is connected to the part of your brain that is used for short-term goals and short-term memory.

Short-term memory is great for remembering seven things, plus or minus two. Seven is the magic number. That's why phone numbers are seven digits. Short-term memory is good to get you out the door, it is not meant to help you make long-term lifestyle changes.

I'll give you an example. Have you ever thought of a phone number and then walked across the room to pick up the phone to dial that number, and while crossing the room, there's there was something on the TV or radio that caught your attention? You just glanced at it for a second before you picked up the phone and then when your fingers went to dial the number you realised it had just disappeared from your head. Has this ever happened to you?

If you can't even make it across the room focusing on the seven digits of a phone number, how are you supposed to make the sort of long-term lifestyle change that is necessary for you to experience permanent weight loss with willpower alone?

When you travel as much as I do, you notice how our airport restaurants and snack bars have high convenience, express foods that aren't healthy at all. Many times I've found myself in search of a quick bite before a flight and unable to find anything other than candies and carbs. Pricey, plastic bagged, nutritionally deficient junk food that is devoid of any nutritive value.

Our daytime schedules are often hectic as well. During the day, most of us rarely get the opportunity to take a lunch hour. Instead, we skip lunch altogether or gulp down a quick sandwich and soft drink while working at the desk. And, when you do go out to a restaurant, you find that they usually have menus listing food with high caloric content that doesn't even provide the nutritional requirements necessary to fuel your body for the rest of the afternoon.

In an attempt to fight the obesity epidemic, New York City now requires that chain restaurants list calories on the menus. Many diners were shocked to discover that a Big Mac and fries comes to over 1,000 calories. Add a shake and it can come to over 2,000 calories, which is the entire recommended daily allowance for the average person.

This isn't a book about cutting calories though. It's about changing your mindset so you don't want to overindulge in the first place. The food you end up eating at those restaurants rarely contributes successfully to that feeling of energy improvement anyway.

Fast food in particular tends to leave people feeling bloated and lethargic, not recharged and revitalized for the rest of the day. The truth is that most restaurant food is not healthy, and it's often served in huge portions that are far more than we actually need to consume.

I haven't even mentioned the nearly endless office parties, birthdays, celebrations, and other events that make it nearly impossible to stay on any kind of a disciplined eating program.

If you're a social person and participate in birthday parties, family dinners, and holiday celebrations you'll probably find that the food choices available to you lie far outside the scope of any diet or nutritional guideline.

At those parties and potlucks everyone brings their favorite foods, and we begin to notice how much those days become filled with temptation after temptation. On days like that it can feel very difficult to discipline yourself with *willpower* alone. The problem is, that it is often considered rude or unsociable not to participate, so we end up eating to make other people feel better even as we make ourselves feel worse. Has this ever happened to you?

Family Dinners

In addition, family dinners have all but disappeared. This is a sad but true reality of the modern world. To paraphrase an old maxim, "The family that eats together, stays together."

Researchers at the University of Minnesota studied 4,682 high school and middle school kids and found that those who ate seven or more meals a week with their parents "had better nutrition... and were less likely to smoke, drink, use marijuana, or show signs of depression." (Project EAT, 2004)

To claim your free gifts (valued at $97) send a blank email to bonus@joshuaseth.com

Today, when families eat, they usually do not do it together. The kids eat while standing around in the kitchen or zoned out in front of the TV with a pizza and coke. The parents may just grab something out of the freezer and throw it into the microwave so they can have a snack while working on the laptop. This has become the typical "family dinner".

For a society that puts so much emphasis on food, we've removed the calm socialization of sitting and slowly eating a healthy meal from the equation for good health and a happy life.

That family meal, which was once lovingly prepared and slowly consumed, full of healthy nutrients used to fortify our bodies, has now transformed into a race of convenience over quality.

Food As Fun

How many events do you celebrate by overindulging in food during the course of a year? Birthdays, holidays, and office parties to name just a few. Coke with cake and ice cream are used as forms of celebration. Nutritional value ZERO. One slice of cake, a glass of coke, and a scoop of ice cream can equal a whole day's worth of non-nutritive calories!

Like in the times of the Roman Empire, when vomitoriums were all the rage, we have once again structured all of our major holidays to revolve around the consumption an impossibly huge meal.

This listing of a typical Thanksgiving dinner could just as easily have been the menu for a bacchanal feast:

- Wine (red and white)

- Mixed drinks (some with sugar and sweet cream)

- Stuffed crab, pigs in a blanket, artichokes soaked in butter, caviar, and jumbo fried shrimp stuffed with cheese and bacon (and those were the appetizers).

- Turkey, ham, roast beef, and a huge broiled lobster tail soaked in garlic butter.

- Three types of stuffing, filled with breads, nuts, butter, fats, fruits and vegetables.

- Breads, rolls, butter, gravies, sweet cranberry sauces.

- Side Dishes: Buttered potatoes, mashed potatoes, and sweet potatoes (all dripping in butter).

- Vegetables: corn (in butter), peas and carrots in butter, creamed spinach, and one or two regular salads with thick creamy dressings.

- Drinks: Coke, Cool-Aid for kids, coffee and tea, after dinner drinks.

- Desserts: pumpkin pie, apple pie, cheese cake, chocolates, puddings, pastries, and cookies.

This is institutionalized engorgement! The ancient Romans would have been proud. One typical Thanksgiving meal can add 3 to 5 pounds, roughly 12 to 15 thousand calories to your eating program *in one day.*

Most people "celebrate" like this many times a year. Don't think so? How about family reunions, Christmas dinner, New Year's Eve, 4th of July picnics, and countless birthday parties, just as a start.

With so many days like these throughout the year, how can willpower stand a chance? It's like being a yo-yo on a string controlled by food and fun.

You can tell yourself that you have control, that you're only going to eat a small amount of food at these big get-togethers, but willpower alone is not enough.

Telling yourself that you have control is one thing, but when your willpower stands up against all of your senses, it's 5 to 1 against. As you walk into the feast, the sights, sounds, smells, and feelings hit you all at once.

The heady aroma brings back memories of celebrations past, and as you begin this emotional journey you begin to salivate at the very thought of things to come.

Then your eyes pop wide open at the sight of all that delectable food, glistening and warm. Steam rising off the platters. Fresh from the oven.

Next, you hear friends and relatives talking about how great last year's event was and how much better this dinner will be.

You walk over to the table and actually touch one of the delicacies. It feels good. It's in your hand now so you taste it, savoring that first bite. You're ready to make a decision. All five senses have voted and it's 5 to 1 against whatever your willpower used to be.

But you remember your promise to yourself. You can't cave this easily. You just got here after all. You muster your strength, your willpower, and lock yourself in the bathroom. You may even be sweating a little from the stress. You wash your face and hands with cool water and compose yourself, letting out a slow deep exhale as you lean against the sink and look yourself in the eye. Get it together! Willpower, remember?

You're ready. You can do this. You emerge back into the swirling rush of the moment and those same smells hit your nose again, causing an instant repeat of the prior sensory episode. Another vote, and this time it's tougher to ignore the results.

Suddenly, there's a hand on your arm, guiding you toward the table. It's your uncle and he's telling you that if you don't EAT, and I mean load your plate up and devour everything in sight until you feel like you're going to explode, then your family will be saying things to you like "What? You don't like Aunt Sophie's Casserole? What's wrong with you?" Or, "Just a little more turkey and stuffing with gravy. You've hardly eaten anything. Don't let all that delicious food go to waste!"

Not eating can be considered rude. The people cooking might feel insulted by your lack of interest in what they've prepared. There's always at least one member of the family who declares, "There's so much food here, and they're starving in other countries. Eat, EAT!"

Society doesn't make it easy to lose weight does it? With rushed schedules, a lack of time for preparation and consumption, and the linking of food with fun, we are continuously under an immense pressure to eat.

We eat too fast. We eat too much. And we eat a lot of foods that have no nutritive value and diminish our health, energy, and well-being.

So don't beat yourself up if you've attempted to use willpower to lose weight in the past and failed. It's not your fault.

It's not you. Willpower's just the wrong tool for the job. You're trying to chop down a tree with a hammer. There are much easier ways to solve your weight issue than by using willpower.

Diets aren't among them.

CHAPTER 4
Why Diets Don't Work

I want you to stop dieting. It's counterproductive. Diets do not work for the vast majority of people who try them. Even those people who do manage to lose weight on a diet tend to put it right back on again (and then some) within a few months. For most people, dieting creates a pattern of weight loss failure and makes it progressively harder to achieve a desirable level of health and fitness. In case you're not convinced, here are seven reasons why you should never diet again.

The Seven Reasons Why Diets Fail

Reason #1

You Feel Like You Are Sacrificing To Lose Weight!

Think of any diet you've ever been on where you couldn't eat one of your favorite foods. For example, let's say the diet you decided to follow would not permit you to have fettucini alfredo, and you really LOVE fettucini alfredo. If you could, you'd have a diet that allowed you to eat fettucini alfredo, morning, noon, and night. But this diet didn't allow it.

So you tell yourself that your diet will only last for a short period of time. Because, if you were able to follow the diet properly, you'd lose weight quickly enough, and then you could eat that pasta again.

The more you try not to think of fettucini alfredo the harder it becomes to avoid it. Suddenly, everywhere you go, you see that fettucini alfredo is not only served, but has become the special of the day, and everyone is eating it in front of you. You're even noticing TV commercials for fettucini alfredo, with that creamy dreamy white cheesy flavor. Fettucini alfredo is everywhere and you can't have any!!

Tell me, how does that make you feel?

Not that good, huh? And when you have a favorite food that you can't eat because of the diet you are on, you always want to eat it more and more.

You begin to feel sorry for yourself because everyone else can eat that delicious food *except you!* Then you start to hate this diet with every bone in your body. It keeps you up at night. Finally you say, "Enough! I can't take this anymore!" and you go out and eat a whole year's supply of that forbidden food in one sitting.

Ugh. Talk about being counter-productive. That process achieves nothing but a negative emotional connection to the idea of losing weight.

Weight loss should not be about sacrifice. It should be a joyful experience. A process to be celebrated. Not a struggle.

How many times have you started a new diet and said to yourself, "Well, I only have to eat this until I lose 10 pounds and then I can go back to eating whatever I ate before.

As long as you want what you cannot have you are pitting your emotions against your capacity for reason. Emotions are stronger than logic. Instead of fighting against yourself, learn how to reprogram your subconscious mind so your thoughts and emotions are in alignment. Then you will both feel and know that you're not sacrificing anything but are instead gaining everything.

Reason #2

The Focus is on the Food, Not YOU.

Diets put your focus on what you cannot have.

Foods you can't have for a day, a week, a month, six months, a year, forever. Diets use your mind to focus on what you're trying to avoid rather than focusing on what is is that you want to gain. This isn't just semantics. It makes all the difference in the world.

Incorrect focus, in this case, would mean that you use your mind to think about the food that you're missing, actually daydreaming that you are eating all those delicious goodies. If you wanted to gain weight rather than lose weight, that would be the perfect way to motivate yourself to do it.

Our lives are governed by certain psychological principles upon which life is based. And one of the most important among them indicates that what you focus on expands. This is often referred to as the Law of Attraction, which is a concept explored in depth in the popular documentary movie "The Secret".

It simply states that whatever you focus on in your mind is what will expand in your life; therefore, if you are focusing on food (or even keeping yourself from it) you will quickly become obsessed with thinking about food, will see food and messages about food all around you, and you will attract more food into your life.

Diets set you up for failure by focusing your attention on exactly what you want to avoid.

Reason #3

Diets Dictate When You Can Eat.

Going back a generation or so, it used to be that the mother of the family would stay at home to take care of the children and the house. She'd provide a healthy, balanced breakfast and dinner for her family. Remember those days? If not imagine 'Father Knows Best'.

Dad would leave for work in the morning after the family breakfast, and be home by 6:00 p.m. During the noon hour, dad would eat the lunch his wife had packed for him. Yes, back then they had established lunchtimes.

At dinner the family would eat together without watching television. They'd actually talk with one another and discuss their day. They knew that 'A family that does dinners together, makes their children winners together'... for life.

You may think that I'm idealizing the past and perhaps I am but the idea of established meals times that involved care and consideration for one another is surely preferable to the current situation in most homes today.

Fast forward to the modern world. Both mom and dad work. About half the time there's only one parent and the kids are left to fend for themselves.

Today we run out of the house in the morning on a cup of coffee or stop by Starbucks for another caffeine fix and a pastry on the way to work.

Work days are now averaging over 10 hours when you factor in travel time. People are eating out more for both lunch and dinner. Fast food seems like a necessity for many time crunched people. Commutes to and from work are long and hard, on heated roads, with heated tempers, and life is more stressful overall.

Who has time for home cooked meals anymore?

Most diets will dictate the time of day you can eat and precisely what you must be eating. With today's hectic lifestyles, it's almost impossible to follow the special eating plan that diets say you must.

Reason #4

Diets Slow Down Your Metabolism.

All diets are restrictive. They restrict what you eat, how much you are allowed to eat, and they dictate at specifically what time you can eat it. That means that when you are hungry the diet may tell you that you cannot eat and you must just deal with it.

When you are hungry, and you don't eat, your body thinks that food is not available and that it's at risk of starving. So it protects you in the only way it knows how, by becoming less efficient at burning whatever fuel you have left. Your metabolism begins to slow down to conserve fuel until food becomes available again.

The truth is that your body doesn't have the conscious intelligence to know that you are intentionally denying it food for its own betterment and you are doing it with all intent and on purpose. It simply responds to the perceived famine in the only way it can.

Your body is a machine which metabolizes food for energy. When there is no food available to burn, it tries to protect you by slowing down the burning of fuel (food). Sooner or later, you lose energy and begin to shut down into groggy, foggy headed sleep, even though it's still the middle of the day. Don't do that to yourself. It's counterproductive to your weight loss goals.

When a perceived famine begins, your metabolism starts taking whatever food it can find in your system and converting it into fat to store away until food becomes available again. That natural process protects us from starving.

This has evolved from the time when our ancestors had to hunt for our food, long before the formation of agrarian societies. In biological time, thousands of years wasn't all that long ago. We are still designed to react to the onset of famine in the way we were programmed to when they were actually part of a typical life cycle.

Food is now readily available everywhere you're likely to be reading this book; however,there's no way for your body to know that if you deny it food when you're hungry.

When you go hungry on purpose, you slow down your metabolism and put yourself into starvation mode. This makes the process of burning calories much more difficult than it needs to be.

Then, when you're done dieting, the increased calories consumed are initially burned at that slower rate. So, when you go back to eating normal food, you have created the ideal conditions for the kind of rapid weight gain that's known as "yo-yoing".

Sound familiar?

Reason #5

Diets Don't Address Emotional Eating

Eating in order to tranquilize negative emotions won't solve the problems that caused those emotions in the first place. It only creates more of a weight issue which in turn causes further emotional problems.

When you eat because you feel bad, or sad, or angry, or lonely, you probably feel worse afterwards. Instead of eating something to feel better, ask yourself what's eating you?

When you eat to feel better, you end up feeling worse because you've let yourself down. You've probably said some rather terrible things to yourself about yourself right after moments such as these.

You might have said to yourself something like "I am going to be fat the rest of my life." or "I hate myself for eating that." or possibly "Great, now I am only going to get fatter and I hate being fat!!"

This negative self-talk creates bad feelings which habit and experience tell you can be quickly tranquilized by eating. Sadly, this becomes a viciously disempowering cycle.

Many people find this sort of situation so disconcerting that they simply give up on the idea of losing weight altogether. This is the typical self-perpetuating process:

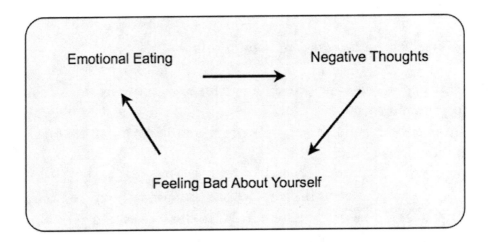

Look at the diagram above and apply it to yourself from a detached, non-emotional perspective. Do you behave in such a way so as to perpetuate this cycle?

Later in this book you are provided with forms that will allow you to track your activities, your thoughts, and your feelings. Notice how you feel when you eat. This can be a crucial step.

Sometimes people subconsciously hold onto their weight for reasons known only to them; emotional reasons that may not be in the forefront of your mind making it difficult to understand what is happening or why it's happening. Nevertheless, these unresolved emotional issues are affecting your life.

Reason #6
Diets Don't Address Fear of Change

Many diets fail simply because they fail to recognize that people can be deeply afraid of the changes that may occur in their lives once they lose weight. For these people, it can be very hard to make behavioral changes to their eating habits without first creating positive associations with what will happen in their lives after the weight is gone.

If a marriage has been sexually dormant as a consequence of being overweight, it's a strong possibility that the loss of weight would bring about the fear change in the relationship. Many people are very resistant to change even though it is the one true constant in the Universe.

Some people don't believe that they have the right to feel good about themselves so they suffer with low self-esteem and a poor body image.

Do you ask yourself "Who am I to be strong, healthy, thin and beautiful? "Well, who are you not to be? Do a checkup on your self-esteem!

Thinking that you are small and insignificant doesn't serve you, and it doesn't serve others. Not living to your full potential is a crime against yourself.

You must allow yourself to grow, to evolve, to become better with every passing day. The only way you can even begin to fulfill your very purpose for living is to first commit to be the best possible You that you can be.

Take a moment right now and imagine the changes will take place in your life when you lose all that excess weight that's been holding you back.

Even if these changes are difficult to accept, are they necessarily bad? Couldn't they potentially lead to a happier life?

You and I both know that most overweight people blame their problems on their weight. Are you one of those blamers or are you actually ready to do something about it?

Do you ever think to yourself, "If I were thin I would get that promotion" or "If I were thin I could get a date" or how about "If I were thin, my spouse would be nicer to me"?

Forget the woulds, coulds, and shoulds. The real fact is, when you lose weight, then your excuse for not getting the promotion, not getting a date, and not being treated well by your spouse will be gone.

When you don't have an easy excuse for the way things are in your life then you have only yourself to blame.

Many people live their lives in the fantasy world of "THE BIG BUT". They make up stories like: "If only I was thin, I could be a beauty queen, BUT because I'm just a little overweight no one respects me."

Of course, it's easy to pretend that your big BUT is getting in the way of getting everything that you want in life.

Isn't it time to get your big BUTT out of the way, and take total responsibility for yourself, your life, and everything in it?

The only way you can ever live life to the fullest is to first commit to being the best possible YOU that you can be.

You are responsible for working hard to get that promotion. *You* are responsible for getting out there and meeting people to get a date. *You* are responsible for deciding if you want to stay with your spouse.

Are you using your weight as an excuse for all the things that you consider wrong with your life?

Perhaps you've always known it, somewhere in the back of your mind, but you chose to ignore it because when your excuse is gone you have make some changes in your life.

Before you can succeed at any weight loss program you must truly believe that you deserve to get the results you want. Then you will welcome the changes that will come as you achieve your weight loss goals.

Reason #7

Diet's Don't Address Self Confidence and Self Esteem

If you don't feel you deserve to lose the weight and lead a better life, then you won't. It's as simple as that. The higher your self-esteem is, the easier it will be for you to achieve your weight loss goals.

Diets restrict what you eat and how much you eat and tell you when you can and cannot eat it. They don't help you to feel like doing something good for yourself in the first place though. If you get discouraged or down on yourself then a diet can't do anything to help you stay on track. For that, you'll need hypnosis.

Every hypnosis session you participate in is an opportunity to enhance your self-esteem. Before you start your self hypnosis sessions, you'll have a chance to do some introspection so you can determine if you have any underlying issues that may have caused you to hold onto weight in the past.

You'll also document your thoughts throughout this program. This is important so you can rapidly get to the root of your overeating problem. You'll discover whether the underlying cause is fear of failure, fear of success, fear of life changes, or something that might transpire once you lose the weight.

Weight issues can simply be the *effects* of low self-esteem that must be transformed into self confidence in order to make behavioral changes easy and successful for you. Don't judge yourself. Simply make honest observations that will help you focus on the areas that need the most improvement.

When you apply *The Weight Loss Hypnosis Solution* in it's entirety, you will be empowered to successfully resolve these issues and achieve success in all areas of your life. Self esteem enhancement is at the root of all personal development.

Now that you know what doesn't work for weight loss, you're ready to learn what does. In the next chapter I'll show you how to use self hypnosis to lose weight using the power of your subconscious mind. I'm excited for you! Let's begin.

CHAPTER 5
The Truth About Hypnosis And Weight Loss

The question I am most often asked when people find out I'm a hypnotist is "Does hypnosis work for weight loss?" Well my answer may surprise you.

You see, a lot of people seem to fall into two camps when it comes to hypnosis and weight loss: there are those who are sceptical about it but are so frustrated with dieting that they're willing to try just about anything to lose weight, and there are those who are just looking for a "you are healed" slap across the head that will magically melt away those unwanted pounds without any effort on their part.

The truth is that while hypnosis is far more effective at losing weight than dieting, without proper nutritional and behavioural education it's nothing more than a feel-good mindset tool.

Anything worth doing in your life takes effort and losing weight is no different. Hypnosis will very effectively put you in a frame of mind that will allow you to make better food choices, but unless you have the proper nutritional and behavioural education it will be of limited value.

For example, if you are an emotional eater (you eat when you're lonely, angry, or depressed) you can easily break this habit with hypnosis. But let's say you're eating because you're actually hungry (a good first step!) and you decide that a soft drink would go well with your meal. In your hypnosis session you became empowered to "eat only when you're hungry and make healthy food choices" (that's actually one of the embedded commands in my 6 CD weight loss hypnosis system). So you ask yourself "Is a diet soft drink a healthier choice than a regular soft drink?"

Without the proper education you may be tempted to think that a diet soft drink is the healthier food choice because it has fewer calories. With some basic nutritional education though, you'll recognise that the aspartame (a sugar substitute found in thousands of "diet" products) in that diet soft drink is far more harmful to your body than the sugar in a regular soda would have been. It may even cause you to gain more weight over time because one of it's documented side effects is increased hunger.

Sure, a glass of water is the best choice of all, but we're all human and the goal is not deprivation but liberation. Freedom from feeling helpless around food because of misinformation and poor internal programming.

Once you understand what good food choices actually are, then you are ready to enjoy all the benefits of weight loss hypnosis. You must attack your weight loss issue from both inside and out: hypnosis works on the inside issues of emotional eating, mindset, and motivation, while proper nutritional and behavioural education works on the outside. Both are necessary for a permanent weight loss solution.

Later in this book I will give you 10 hypnotic weight loss suggestions that you can use to achieve your goals. Each of these behaviour modification exercises are actually hypnotic suggestions that will subconsciously reprogram your eating habits so you'll lose weight without even thinking about it. First though it's important to understand exactly what hypnosis is and how it works.

What Is Hypnosis?

Since the beginning of recorded history there have been examples of hypnosis, including tribal ceremonies of early humans.

One of the earliest written records describing hypnosis was found in an ancient Egyptian tomb, written on papyrus, and was 3500 years old. It is known that the Egyptians, Greeks and Romans all used hypnosis for medical and religious purposes.

To help develop his theories on psychoanalysis, Sigmund Freud used hypnosis with his patients to gain information from them that they might otherwise have been resistant to reveal.

World War I and World War II saw the use of hypnosis as an anesthetic when supplies were low, and also for the treatment of soldiers with combat neurosis, which today is called post-traumatic stress disorder.

In terms of medical use, in 1892 the British Medical Association (BMA) formally recognized that hypnosis had applications in modern medicine.

Later in 1958, the American Medical Association (AMA) declared hypnosis was a useful medical tool.

In laboratory settings, researchers have used hypnosis to create false memories, hallucinations, compulsions, and alternative behaviors so that they could be studied, catalogued, and analyzed.

One of the tools used in the medical field is called a positron emission tomography (PET) scan. It records an image of the brain. It has been used to prove that hypnosis produces a very specific pattern of activity within the brain.

PET scans on those in hypnotic states demonstrate an increased blood flow in the right anterior cingulate cortex. This suggests that there are internal focus scenarios occurring and that this focused brain activity is very different from what occurs in normal waking states.

Brain Wave Classifications

There are four classifications of brain wave rhythms. They are beta, alpha, theta and delta.

Beta waves occur during the normal waking consciousness state. As you read this book, you are probably in beta. Beta is a state where you are wide awake and aware of your surroundings.

Alpha waves are a slower brainwave pattern found when people relax, listen to music, or meditate.

Theta waves are present just before you fall asleep and after you awaken from a deep sleep. In this state you may day dream or "zone out". Theta waves are present during the hypnotized trance state.

Delta waves occur during deep sleep. Delta waves allow you to rest and rejuvenate.

The Science Behind Hypnosis

By using the PET scan scientists have made some exciting discoveries regarding hypnosis. For instance, many people had assumed that hypnosis was simply enhanced imagination. This is now known not to be true.

Although it is a common misconception, it has been proven by medical science that there is no relationship between hypnosis and imagination.

Many people experience auditory and visual hallucinations while they are in a hypnotic trance. That's why people sometimes assume a connection between imagination and hypnosis.

With the PET scan, brain researchers have determined that there are different regions of the brain that are activated during hypnosis than are activated when using the imagination alone.

They determined that when a person imagines a sound, that activity is located in a specific region of the brain, and when that same person experiences a hypnotic hallucination, the brain activity occurs somewhere totally different.

Henry Szechtman and his staff at McMaster University in Ontario, Canada used a PET scan to record the brain activity of hypnotized individuals who imagined a scene and then who experienced a hallucination.

They found that when imagining a sound it is experienced internally; however, when hallucinating a sound in hypnosis, it is experienced as though it came from an external source.

Then, they attempted to isolate the area of the brain responsible for this different brain response pattern in hypnosis while doing a PET scan.

Eight subjects where studied by Szechtman and his colleagues during a hallucinationatory session.

During the session, each person heard the exact same audio sample while the PET scanner recorded the activity. Their brain activity was observed during four segments:

- While they were listening in their normal waking state.

- While they simply rested and heard the audio sample.

- While they just imagined hearing the audio sample.

- While they were in a hypnotic trance state responding to a suggestion to hallucinate the audio sample, although it was not actually playing.

This research revealed that the region of the brain called the right anterior cingulate cortex was every bit as active while hallucinating as it was when the test subjects were actually hearing the stimulus.

In comparison, the right anterior cingulate cortex was not active while the volunteers were simply imagining that they heard the audio sample.

Hypnosis had completely deceived that area of the brain into registering the hallucinated voice as genuine.

The Power Of Hypnosis

Some of the earliest trials of clinical hypnosis were for the treatment of pain and medical conditions in the US military. These case histories are well documented from all around the world.

Back in 1969, Thomas H. McGlashan and his colleagues at the University of Pennsylvania discovered that for lower-level scale hypnotizable subjects, hypnosis was as useful in reducing pain as a sugar pill that they had been instructed was a powerful painkiller. But, those subjects who were highly hypnotizable received three times the amount of benefit from hypnosis as from the placebo pills.

At the University of Montreal in 1997, Pierre Rainville studied the brain response during hypnotic pain relief. The purpose of the study was to locate the areas of the brain that were associated with suffering as part of pain, as separate from its sensory aspects.

That study, while using the PET scans, demonstrated on film that hypnosis reduced the activity of the anterior cingulate cortex (the area known to be involved with pain). It also showed that it was not a factor in the activity of the somatosensory cortex (where the pain sensations are processed).

The National Institutes of Health Technology assessment panel, in 1996 judged hypnosis to be a valuable tool for alleviating pain from cancer and other chronic conditions.

In the International Journal of Clinical and Experimental Hypnosis, a study revealed that hypnotic suggestions relieved 75 percent of the pain for 933 subjects in a total of 27 different experiments.

All of this tends to indicate, that pain relief can easily be accomplished with the help of hypnotic suggestion. It verifies that hypnotic control of pain is a valuable and important life tool. In some cases, the degree of hypnotic relief exceeded the relief provided by use of morphine.

Can Hypnosis Be Faked?

Many people wonder, "How do you know if people are really hypnotized? Couldn't they just fake it?" Of course people *try* to fake hypnosis, but that's very simple for a trained hypnotist to recognize.

Two studies worth noting regard attempts to fake the hypnotic trance state. The first took place in 1971 at the University of Pennsylvania by Frederick Evans and Martin T. Orne. This study contrasted the reactions of two different groups of subjects. One was made up of people who were hypnotized and the other was made up of people that were told to pretend that were hypnotized.

An experimenter was instructed to conduct a hypnotic procedure that, unknown to him, would be interrupted by a pre-arranged power failure.

Naturally, the experimenter would leave the room to investigate the power failure. The subjects who were pretending immediately came out of the fake hypnotic state and began reacting to the power outage.

In contrast, the participants who were hypnotized, awakened from hypnosis slowly and with some difficulty.

In another study, by Taru Kinnunen, Harold S. Zamansky and their colleagues at Northeastern University. They used a polygraph (lie detector) to measure the response of hypnotized subjects and those subjects faking hypnosis.

While faking hypnosis, the lie detector revealed the responses as it would with anyone.

However, when the lie detector was used on the hypnotized subjects, it could not distinguish truth from lies.

When a hypnotized person is given suggestions, their full physiological system reacts appropriately and supports those suggestions as their own personal truth.

There seems to be no internal distinction between real or suggested events while a subject is in a hypnotic trance.

For high achievers, this information comes as no surprise Successful individuals have been using hypnosis for years to increase their mental skills, enhance their overall performance, and increase their success in life.

Hypnosis has been used by countless athletes, sales people, managers, executives and students to achieve extraordinary results in their fields.

Can I Be Hypnotized?

"Hypnosis sounds great, but can I be hypnotized? I'm not sure I can. I'm a very stubborn person, plus I don't have a good attention span, and I hate to give up control to anyone else."

These are common concerns, so it may surprise you to know that you've already experienced hypnosis several times a day, every single day of your life. Hypnosis is a natural state of mind.

All hypnosis is really self hypnosis.

A skilled hypnotist can act as a guide to achieving and maintaining theta state and can supply well crafted suggestions to use while you are there but ultimately it's an internal process and therefore you do it to yourself.

Hypnosis is a skill that you can develop because it's a state of mind you slip in and out of already.

Have you ever been completely immersed in something to the exclusion of everything else? That is a natural trance state.

Examples of this occur while watching a movie and becoming transfixed in the plot, while driving and being hypnotized by the road ahead, or while working intently and finding that the last four hours have flown by without being consciously aware of it.

Hypnosis occurs when you're reading a book and so wrapped up in it that you don't even notice it when someone talks to you.

Have you ever been surprised or "woken" from that state of mind and then had to have the person repeat what they just said? We all experience this hypnotic trance state naturally and with some regularity throughout the day.

So yes, you can be hypnotised. If you read this page over more than once perhaps you already are!

Fear Based Worries

By now, I hope you've begun to realize, that you are not signing a pact with the devil and that hypnosis is not witchcraft, manipulation, or magic. It is simply a tool that allows you to tap into the power of your mind to achieve success in all areas of your life.

Fear-based thoughts about hypnosis began almost 180 years ago in England, when surgeon James Braid, MD, who was successful in treatment of a crippling children's disorder, began to research and use hypnosis with his patients.

A nearby church, without cause or provocation, began attacks on this doctor who saved and transformed children's lives. Braid responded by writing a treatise which became a book. In the book he attempted to reason with these superstitious people who refused to view, review, read, or see hypnosis in action as part of medical treatment. Because of Dr. Braid's work, the use of hypnosis was accepted in England about a century before it was accepted in the United States. Dr. James Braid is considered the founder of modern medical hypnosis.

Fear regarding hypnosis was most often spread by religions, who had no experience with the science. Recently, religion and science have come to terms with the use of hypnosis, and a segment of Christian therapies now includes Christian hypnosis.

Hypnosis has worked for millions of people for thousands of years, became a science over 150 years ago, is recognized by all major medical and psychiatric associations around the world and has been shown to be effective in the treatment of diseases and disorders.

There is no reason to fear any negative side effects from the use of hypnosis. I am personally unaware of any documented negative side effects ever resulting from hypnosis. Just superstitions, such as "getting stuck in a trance", which is impossible. You can no more get stuck in a trance than you can get stuck asleep.

What is typical, is that people who were previously fearful of hypnosis, consistently indicate how positively impacted they have been from the experience once they realize that it's simply a very effective way to direct your internal focus toward the achievement of your goals.

What Do I Need To Do To Be Hypnotized?

All you need to be hypnotized is a willingness to relax and focus on the positive suggestions that you will be receiving.

Another requirement is that you have a minimum IQ level of 60, but since you've read this far I think you've got that one covered.

The key here is to relax. If you are not willing to relax, then you'll have trouble focusing. Both are necessary in order to achieve hypnosis. In fact, "focused relaxation" is one definition for hypnosis.

The more you practice self-hypnosis the easier it becomes for you to enter the hypnotic trance state.

Going Into Hypnosis

You can enter a hypnotic state anywhere you desire, no matter what sounds surround you, whether there's daylight, bright light, or no light. The process is easy and it's called an induction.

Sometimes hypnotists will utilize soothing sounds or even music because it makes the hypnotic state easier to achieve and more satisfying for the subject.

How Does Hypnosis Work?

Hypnosis works for behavior change (weight loss, smoking cessation, etc.) by communicating with your subconscious mind through the use of suggestion. To fully understand how hypnosis bypasses your critical faculties to get these suggestions easily accepted, it's important to understand the differences between your conscious and subconscious states of mind.

Do you remember the last time you drove your vehicle? Was it to go to work, or to go shopping, or run an errand? Remember your last trip.

Do you recall the details of that ride? Most people can't. You only really consciously drive your vehicle when you're first learning. Driving is done at an unconscious level. You don't say to yourself "Now I have to put the key in the starter, turn the key, put my seat beat on, put the vehicle in gear, release the parking brake, check over my left shoulder for oncoming traffic, check the rear view mirror, put my turn signal on to turn left, turn the steering wheel, release the steering wheel and straighten the vehicle, and now press on the gas peddle to go straight ahead" and so on.

Driving is a learned, habitual activity. Your subconscious is aware of everything that is happening, but because it's a habit you are consciously thinking about other things: what you still need to do, what you want to watch on TV later in the evening, or what you wished you would have said or done earlier in the day.

We all shift from conscious to subconscious states of mind without thought or effort.

Take this simple test:

I fly a
a kite everyday

What did you see? Your selective conscious mind would probably have you focus on just the letters of the sentence structure. I'm certain you also saw the book you're holding, possibly the floor beneath it, and perhaps the furniture that is beside you.

Consciously, you became very selective of what your mind was processing. Subconsciously, your awareness was fully absorbed by all these other factors. There were other stimuli as well.

Once directed consciously, you may have become aware of the sounds in the room around you, or of the temperature, or the quality of the light.

More than likely while you were taking that simple test these elements were not even in your consciousness. By the way, did you read the word "a" twice in the above sentence?

Perception dictates reality.

Hypnosis For Stress Management

Feel stressed? Don't worry, everyone feels stress from time to time.

Many stress management programs exist. The best, in my opinion utilize self-hypnosis to regulate, reduce, and convert unhealthy stress to it's positive form, known as eustress. Eustress is a motivating energy that can convert debilitating distress into a positive force that can propel you to the heights of success. Hypnosis is a great way to facilitate that process so you can reach your weight loss goals. It's important to learn how to manage your stress well because when most people feel stressed out they eat in order to feel better.

I've encountered many people who think that constant stress is unavoidable. They typically say to me, "The only time I can turn things off in my head is when I sleep."

Ironically, while you're sleeping, you're really not turning anything off at all. Instead, you're turning other things on.

To claim your free gifts (valued at $97) send a blank email to bonus@joshuaseth.com

You are adjusting your state of awareness. You have entered a delta level of brain wave activity which involves rejuvenating yourself physically while your subconscious goes right on working during sleep.

Let me ask you, have you ever had a challenge that you could not resolve? Or have you ever found yourself trying to remember the answer to a question that you know you knew five minutes earlier, but cannot recall now?

If this has ever happened to you, the answer probably returned to your your conscious awareness as soon as you stopped trying to remember it.

Maybe you woke up this morning and had it on the tip of your tongue. As soon as you took your attention off thinking about it and focused on other things, your subconscious took over and delivered exactly the information you needed.

Subconscious Solutions

The other day I was watching a documentary on musicians. They interviewed a number of songwriters who spoke about how they had awoken in the middle of the night and written the biggest hit of their career. None of them were consciously aware of it until the next morning when they found the composition sitting next to the bed.

It was like that with Albert Einstein, who had a vision of walking on a sunbeam and discovering the theory of relativity. And also with Thomas Edison's discovery for the workings of a light bulb during his sleep.

In actuality the subconscious never sleeps, it continues taking care of the requirements for the physical body and it sends messages, in the form of dreams, to solve the problems of your life.

Your subconscious is your fully automatic problem-solving machine, and it's designed to give you exactly what you want, when you know how to instruct it appropriately. The most effective way to instruct your subconscious mind to give you what you want in life is with hypnosis.

How It Feels To Be Hypnotized

I'm sure you've seen those zombie-like characters in the movies and on TV that are supposedly in some form of a trance.

This is one of the most common misconceptions about hypnosis.

These zombie like depictions have given people the impression that there's a loss of control during hypnosis. This couldn't be farther from the truth. You're always in control.

When you are in a hypnotic trance state, you are in more control than during your normal waking state. During hypnosis your blood flow is increased in the right anterior cingulate cortex. This would tend to suggest that there is an internal focus, not a complete release of control. As you become internally focused, your surrounding environment becomes less important and less significant to you.

By the way, if for any reason there was an emergency or your attention was needed, you would automatically and immediately awaken yourself to respond appropriately to the situation at hand. After all, you're not knocked out or unconscious, you're in your subconscious and still able to respond to external stimuli.

Controlled Level Of Relaxation

When you are in a controlled hypnotic state of trance, your body will typically experience deep levels of relaxation. You may look as if you are asleep but the biological state of trance is very different from sleep.

You may be slumped over in relaxation but while your body is relaxed your mind will be alert and aware. You will perceive all of the suggestions that you are receiving. Hypnosis is definitively NOT what is normally thought of as sleep.

In this state of mind, external distractions become irrelevant because your focus is on the suggestions that you are receiving.

While you are in hypnosis, your breathing will become rhythmic and regular. You may even experience a distortion of your sense of time. You'll feel like you've been under for just a few minutes, even if it's been over an hour.

Hypnosis And Weight Loss

There have been numerous scientific studies that have verified the effectiveness of hypnosis when applied to weight loss. In 1996, the Journal of Consulting and Clinical Psychology analyzed five of these weight loss studies and reported that the " ... weight loss reported in the five studies indicates that hypnosis can more than double the effects of traditional weight loss approaches."

When you tap into the power of your subconscious mind to influence your eating habits and release your emotional reliance on food then you can eat what you want without depriving yourself of anything. This is the essence of why hypnosis works for weight loss even when diets and willpower fail.

Now that you know what hypnosis is and how effectively it can be used for losing weight, let's make sure the diet industry doesn't sneak in and sabotage your progress!

CHAPTER 6
How Diet Foods Are Making You Fatter

If I were to tell you it's not your fault, you're not to blame for being overweight, would you believe me? If I asked you why you blame yourself for having overwhelming cravings or puzzling yo-yo weight fluctuations, what would you tell me?

The truth is it's not your fault! Society has already judged you and said that if you're not as thin as a cover girl model – you're too heavy! And because of how you feel as a result of this societal judgment, you've gone and tried every diet that's ever been discovered without real long-lasting success.

Many people actually have adverse reactions to the chemicals found in diet foods. You may have undiagnosed allergies or sensitivities to the chemicals that are being used in food today that you are not even aware of. Perfume, hair spray, fabric softener, car exhaust, pesticides, smog, wheat, sugar, second hand smoke and exposure to various foods or chemicals can all trigger cravings, even binges, and result in weight gain.

Look for potential connections between changes in your weight and the kinds of food you eat (instead of being focused on how much you eat) also take note of when and where cravings, uncontrollable hunger and binges occur. This is one of the reasons you have been given a Food Diary as a bonus with this book. You'll get a downloadable version, so you can print out as many copies as you need, when you sign up at www.joshuaseth.com/bonus. Also pay attention to any changes you may have in moods or thoughts such as: anger, depression, crying, irritability, and inability to concentrate and think clearly.

The same substances that cause weight gain and cravings can also create symptoms that appear to be psychological, but are really a result of sensitivity to a food or chemical.

In my weight loss hypnosis sessions I repeatedly implant the suggestion to "make healthy food choices", but how are you supposed to know what's healthy when deadly poisons are labeled as sugar-free "diet food"?

I'm specifically talking about the chemical food additive Aspartame, which is a sugar substitute found in over 6,000 food products.

Why Am I Writing About A Sugar Substitute?

After all, I'm a hypnotist not a nutritionist. Well it's because your mind and your body work together. Your behavior is a result of your thinking. Nutritional education alone won't help you lose weight if you're still emotionally addicted to certain foods. And while Hypnosis can easily break you of those food cravings, you also need to know what constitutes healthy eating habits.

As the tens of thousands of people who have attended my Hypnosis for Weight Loss Seminars or listened to my Weight Loss Hypnosis CDs know, all the motivation and good intentions in the world won't help you lose weight if you then make poor eating choices.

Unfortunately, because of improper education and deceptive labeling practices on the part of the diet industry, people often think they're making healthy eating choices by substituting sugar with the powder in those colorful little packets. The truth is that artificial sugar substitutes are not healthy, they're not safe, and they're actually making you fatter.

The Truth About Aspartame

Aspartame is the artificial sweetener found in thousands of diet foods. It's also marketed as a sugar substitute under the names "Equal" and "NutraSweet". The next time you reach for a diet soda or sugar-free chewing gum, check the list of ingredients, you'll probably find that it contains Aspartame.

It's absolutely mind-blowing to me that this stuff is still legal, when you consider that the FDA itself has reported that Aspartame accounts for 75% of all complaints of adverse reactions to our food supply.

Just because the FDA approves the use of a chemical additive doesn't mean it's safe (Saccharine anyone? How about some Fen-phen?) As you digest Aspartame it breaks down into several other chemicals as it makes it's way through your body. Guess what it breaks down into...

- Methanol (which is also known as wood alcohol and is a deadly poison)

- Formaldehyde (a deadly neurotoxin in the same class as cyanide and arsenic)

- Free Form Aspartic Acid (which has been linked to serious neurological disorders)

- Phenylalanine (decreases serotonin which can cause mood swings and depression)

Not surprisingly, the presence of this chemical poison in your body results in a number of side effects. I won't list some of the more sensational (and therefore controversial) side effects. I'll just stick with some of the garden variety side effects. I think they'll more than make the point.

To claim your free gifts (valued at $97) send a blank email to bonus@joshuaseth.com

Some Of The MANY Reported Side Effects Of Aspartame Are:

- Headaches

- Dizziness

- Depression

- Fatigue

- Anxiety

- Irritability

- Hair Loss

- Hearing Loss

- Memory Loss

- Vision Problems

- Sleep Problems

- Abdominal Pain

- Weight Gain

Let's just address that last side effect for now: Weight Gain.

How Does Aspartame Cause Weight Gain

You probably think you're doing something proactive to reduce your weight and increase your health when you drink a diet soda because it has less calories than a regular soda, right?

The reality though is that the Aspartame in that drink has dozens of very unhealthy side effects, not the least of which is that it increases your appetite.

So even though you're taking in fewer calories by drinking that diet soda, you're going to start feeling hungry and end up consuming even more calories from other foods than you would have in the first place. Does that make sense? Not if you want to lose weight.

The bottom line is: You're not really reducing your overall caloric intake when you drink that Diet Coke because it's going to make you hungry.

What About All Those Other Symptoms?

Most people just take a pill to treat the symptoms and remain unaware of the cause. Symptoms compound though and become worse over time. The next thing you know, you're taking even more pills which cause even more side effects. American's are now taking so much medication that they can't even absorb it all and are peeing it back out into what becomes our drinking water (but that's a subject for another book).

I'm not saying that if you suffer from some of these symptoms it's necessarily because of Aspartame. I am saying that you can easily eliminate one of the causes of all of these symptoms at once. So why not do it?

Is There A Debate About Aspartame Side Effects?

Yes. Have you noticed that whenever a product that generates billions of dollars in profits is found to be unsafe, there's a debate about it? Big corporations don't just give those products up without a fight. They sponsor their own research and have their own agendas.

No one seems to be debating if Aspartame is bad for you. They're just debating about the severity of the side effects and how much exposure to the stuff will produce them.

Why take the risk? What's the upside? A few less calories? You know what, if you really want a Coke then just have a Coke. Don't make yourself nuts about all this stuff.

Sure it's better not to have ANY soft drinks at all, but the objective is better health, not food fascism. Drink water whenever possible. Limit the amount of soft drinks you consume. And when you do have soda don't have a "diet soda". Simple.

Make that one behavioral change on the outside while using self hypnosis to reduce your stress and your food cravings on the inside and you will create the conditions for better health and easy weight loss.

A Word About Splenda

Splenda, which is actually the synthetic chemical Sucralose. It's basically chlorinated sugar. It's not a naturally occurring substance, It's undergone very little human testing. And it's being used as a sugar substitute in thousands of diet foods.

It's yet another example of the diet industry telling people that they can have something for nothing. You can NEVER (and I use that word very rarely, as Socrates cautions against it) never have something for nothing in this life. You'll always pay some sort of a price for it.

You want sugar, it comes with calories. You want chemical substitutes, they come with side effects. You want neither calories nor chemicals, you don't get to eat sweet foods.

The choice is yours. Hopefully this information will at least empower your decision making process. Personally, I like local honey!

CHAPTER 7
Start With The End In Mind

Through my live seminars I've been able to help thousands of people discover that they don't ever have to starve themselves to lose weight. The truth is that you can, in fact, still eat all the foods you love while being more satisfied by eating less of them.

Boy was I was lucky. I grew up practicing these principles naturally because my father's a psychologist and a hypnotherapist and my mother has so many psychological credentials after her name that it looks like alphabet soup!

I was fortunate to have grown up all my life, learning and practicing the very principles outlined in this book. To me, it's just a way of life and it wasn't until after I began working with other people, helping them reach their weight loss goals, that I realized that these principles and techniques weren't as common to everyone as I'd thought!

Believe You Can Succeed

It was then that I realized what the problem was: that I could tell you something absolutely true, like "it's important that you truly imagine yourself as a thin person before you can consistently take the steps necessary to become one". You can hear it and know that it's true. Yet there's probably this little voice in your head that pipes in and says "yeah but..."

As in "yeah, but I've got so much weight to lose" or "yeah, but I've been overweight for so long".

This 'yeah, but' is your conscious mind messing with you! It's up there playing devil's advocate, stopping you before you've even started. You must turn that self-defeating, second-guessing, constantly criticizing part of your mind off. Once you do this, you can achieve your goals more effectively. In fact, through hypnosis, that little voice inside of you transforms to become your own cheerleading squad saying "YES, I can do this!"

I know that's easier said than done. Yet, believing in your own ability to succeed makes it easier for you to accomplish your weight loss goals. And, it's also one of the reasons that hypnosis works so well.

During hypnosis, that self-conscious part of your brain is soothingly put to "sleep" so that your unconscious mind can become more fully aware and accepting of the suggestions. Because it easily accepts them, it can automatically apply these suggestions to your behavior so you can enjoy the positive results.

While you are in a state of hypnosis, you'll begin to imagine yourself as a thin person and really visualize yourself as your ideal self staring back at you in the mirror of your mind.

You will actually hear and feel and accept my positive words of encouragement, without negatively critiquing yourself into becoming inactive.

Beyond this, you'll begin to feel successful, happy, and healthy because you're improving yourself every single day.

In this way you will discover that you're quickly and easily losing the excess weight that's been dragging you down. And you'll begin to enjoy all the fun and freedom that comes with being the new, thinner you.

CHAPTER 8
The Secret And You

There's a documentary movie called "The Secret" that got a ton of attention in the past few years. Turns out that the secret they're referring to is a universal principle called The Law of Attraction, which simply states that 'Whatever you focus on expands.'

The Law of Attraction works by magnetizing into your life the manifestation of whatever you've focused upon, imagined clearly, and infused with feeling. Over time, you will begin to live the reality of that emotionally charged focus.

People who have studied and applied the Law of Attraction find that it empowers them to attract what they want; wealth where there was poverty, health where there was illness, and happiness where there was sadness. It can also attract a healthy, lean, and attractive body where there had been an out of shape body before.

Now, this is not a new psychological principle. Mother Theresa was famously quoted as saying she would never be a part of any anti-war rally because it's still focused on war, she'd only be a part of a pro-peace rally because it's focused on the outcome she wants.

So, Mother Theresa was stating in her own way the same principle now known as the Law of Attraction. She'd only focus on the outcome she wanted so as to create more of it.

Here's how it relates to weight loss: when you become focused on seeing yourself as fit, trim, healthy, and already at your goal weight, you will begin to manifest that internal reality externally. Start with the end in mind and focus on the outcome you desire. Not the pounds you want to lose but the lifestyle you want to gain.

Careful though, there can be a philosophical conflict when you want to use the Law of Attraction to focus on "losing weight" because you are actually creating a focus on the excess weight that must be lost. According to the Law of Attraction, in order for you be able to lose weight there must be an acceptance, rather than resistance, and you must accept that there simply is too much weight. If you accept that there is too much weight, you're not seeing the end result of a thin body. Therefore it will not work!

According to the Law of Attraction, by focusing on losing weight, you are actually focusing on the problem (too much weight), rather than the desired outcome (being fit and healthy and full of energy). This is where many people get confused in their attempts to use the Law of Attraction everywhere to effect differences in their lives.

You do not want to put your focus on weight and loss and food and keeping yourself from it. Instead, turn your focus toward manifesting the outcome you desire: a slim, fit, and attractive body.

Therefore, in your self hypnosis sessions (included at the end of this book) you'll notice that the suggestions don't focus on weight loss, they focus instead on becoming the person you desire to be. This shift in focus from losing weight to gaining the body you desire can make all the difference in the world.

Understand The Law Clearly

Now that you understand how the Law of Attraction works, reframe what you want. Instead of trying to lose weight, focus instead on gaining fitness.

To accomplish this, you must create a mental image of your healthy body in your mind's eye. You must see the results in your imagination and anchor it with positive emotion. Accept it as an already accomplished fact that you are simply reflecting on and enjoying in your mind.

Focus On What You Want

Remember that what you focus on expands. If you're constantly focused on the food that you're keeping yourself away from, that's a negative focus. If you keep that focus, you'll develop an obsession.

Instead, focus on seeing yourself as you wish to be.

'But I Just Can't Imagine Myself As Thin'

When an overweight person says they cannot visualize themselves with a perfect, healthy, body that's when they cannot attract it. And psychologists tell us that the more we weigh, the harder it is to visualize ourselves at the perfect weight.

So, if you have 100 or more pounds to lose, and you've been that heavy for most of your life, and you have a difficulty seeing yourself slim and trim, STOP. Take a deep breath and begin to improve your ability to visualize and imagine. This is one of the areas where hypnosis will help. By guiding you through this imaginative process so you can clearly see what you would look like as a thin person and believe it is possible for you to manifest that reality in your life. Here's a simple technique to get you started:

Start Small

If you're in this *can't imagine* category, don't try to see the perfect body just yet. Instead choose a body a few steps closer to being perfectly healthy and slender. See yourself with 1/3 or ½ of the weight gone. Imagine something that you can easily visualize. When you've met that first goal, you can then adjust your imaging until you obtain the ideal body you really want.

Once you can visualize your new ideal body, you'll want to focus your attention on it as often as you can. And while you are focusing on your new physique, begin to feel some positive emotions. Feel your new body and see yourself dancing, running, jumping, playing and having a GREAT life. Associate positive emotions with the image of the new you.

Energize It!

The more energy and excitement you can generate around having this new body, the faster it will arrive. Dance, swim, bicycle, exercise, live life with a passion and enjoy creating that fantastic energy that charges you up and makes you feel great. Infuse that image of the new ideal body with your face and a radiant, abundant energy... in your mind, see it every day!

You must be able to see yourself, and simultaneously believe that you are becoming your ideal self, to begin the series of behavioral changes that will create that slim, ideal you.

Keep Your Eye On The Goal

In order for this process to work optimally... You must start with the end in mind, quite literally. In hypnotic terms, this is the concept called 'fait accompli' from the French hypnotists and doctors studying it in the 1800's. It means that the hypnosis script included the words ... 'it is already an accomplished fact...'

The use of the fait accompli dialogue on the mind while it is hypnotized convinces the subconscious that the desired outcome already exists, therefore it cannot be otherwise.

Because two opposing concepts cannot exist in the same mind at the same time, you'll physically begin to gravitate toward and manifest into your new life the accomplished fact of having a healthy, thin, and fit body. You'll naturally begin to adopt the behaviors that go along with your new mindset.

CHAPTER 9
Emotional Eating

Self esteem, stress and weight are all interconnected. If your stress is high it's hard to lose weight because most people turn to food as a form of control and comfort. If your self esteem is low it's hard to lose weight because you're not in a state of mind that is conducive to self improvement.

When you eat to feel better it's called "emotional eating". It's a crutch I'm going to kick out from under you before we're done so you can stand on your own two feet and be proud of who you are.

Have you ever noticed that people who are relatively stress-free are often those with the highest levels of self esteem? They have a quiet self-assurance that is independent of any external situation. They don't care if other people like them or not, and they have no need for the approval of others because they already approve of themselves.

Their management of stress seems to come naturally as part of their way of living. Self esteem isn't really much of an issue for them either. Many people admire and like to be around individuals who exude self confidence. It's sexy.

As we evolve towards that heightened level of self esteem, there is less need to control other people or situations and therefore less stress in our lives.

To claim your free gifts (valued at $97) visit www.joshuaseth.com/bonus

When you have a sense of inner confidence, where there is no need for you to impress anyone but yourself, stress management becomes effortless.

The way you feel about yourself impacts your overall happiness. The less stress you feel, the more potential you will have to live a balanced life so you won't indulge in unhealthy eating habits in the first place.

If you trust your ability to handle whatever stresses come along in life, you'll be more likely to interpret difficult situations as challenges to grow from, rather than as problems to overcome.

If you don't trust your own ability to handle life's little surprises, then you'll be more likely to perceive the world around you as threatening and stress provoking.

A major influence on a your self esteem is your own 'self talk', which is simply the way you talk to yourself, the way you interpret things, and the way you filter information about your life.

A thinking style that is habitually negative can perpetuate a negative viewpoint of yourself and of life in general.

If you've got a poor self image, that is easy to change with self hypnosis. Without a good self image you may try to use willpower to control food, eating, or weight in order to achieve a sense of personal control.

If you've had a problem with excess, it's likely to have impacted your self esteem. You may have experienced some form of failure due to a yo-yo dieting cycle, embarrassment, shame, or a lack of confidence from negative social responses to and judgments about your weight.

Don't eat to make yourself feel better. Don't eat just because it's cheap or it's fast or it's convenient. Don't eat just because food is on your plate and you feel compelled to finish it.

Eat because you're hungry and your body needs to replenish itself and restore it's energy. Learn to reconnect your mind with your body. Learn what it's like to feel satisfied after a meal instead of stuffed full to bursting.

Take back your life.

The lack of health and energy you see all around you isn't normal; it's the sad result of the disconnection of our minds from our bodies and our bodies from our true selves. We've allowed other people to tell us how we should look, act, and feel about ourselves. We've been trained to think that following diets and counting calories are the roadmaps to fitness and good health. It's much more simple than that.

Your Life Reflects Your Thinking

Your mind and body are linked together within the person that is you. When you make the commitment to improve your life in any one area you inevitably begin to address all the other areas too.

Permanent weight loss is difficult to achieve without implementing stress reduction techniques as well. Permanent stress reduction is a real challenge to maintain without improving your self esteem so you feel that you deserve to live a better quality of life. To really make meaningful changes in any one area of your life it requires a commitment to improving your whole life.

To claim your free gifts (valued at $97) send a blank email to bonus@joshuaseth.com

Your mind and your body are connected after all, so to make physical changes that you desire you must also make mental changes. Everything begins with thought. Your thinking determines your beliefs, your attitudes, your expectations, and ultimately your outcomes.

Your whole life is a reflection of your thinking up until now. So if you want to change and improve your future in any way all you really need to do is commit to changing the way you think.

This realization is simple but profound. It doesn't require research and education, merely self refection, personal responsibility, and a commitment to change.

On the following page is an exercise to help you incorporate this belief system into your thinking.

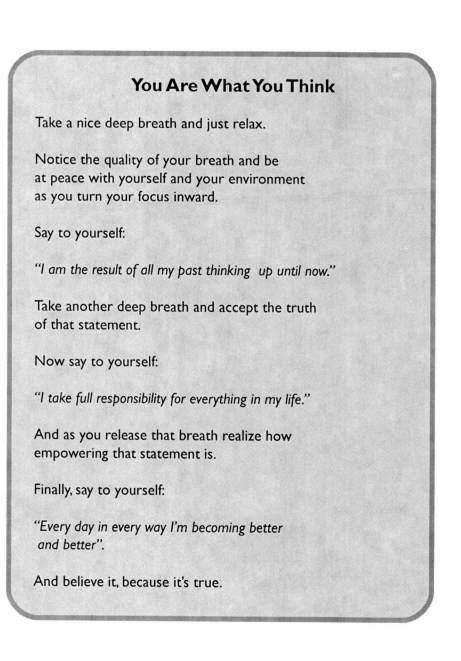

You Are What You Think

Take a nice deep breath and just relax.

Notice the quality of your breath and be
at peace with yourself and your environment
as you turn your focus inward.

Say to yourself:

"I am the result of all my past thinking up until now."

Take another deep breath and accept the truth
of that statement.

Now say to yourself:

"I take full responsibility for everything in my life."

And as you release that breath realize how
empowering that statement is.

Finally, say to yourself:

*"Every day in every way I'm becoming better
and better".*

And believe it, because it's true.

CHAPTER 10
Your Mind Body Connection

Our well-designed physical machine operates automatically through a computerized brain.

When you examine the human body, or any part of it, through an electron microscope, you will discover that the apparent physical organs are really only atoms in motion. We are atomic, that means that we are Energy!

This statement is supported by the laws of physics. This is a Universe of energy, and what we call physical things are simply massive amounts of energy. That includes the world and everything in it. Under a microscope, your car, your home, your office, your computer are all just atoms – energy.

Our minds are also made up of energy. There are two very distinct parts to the human mind, the conscious and the subconscious.

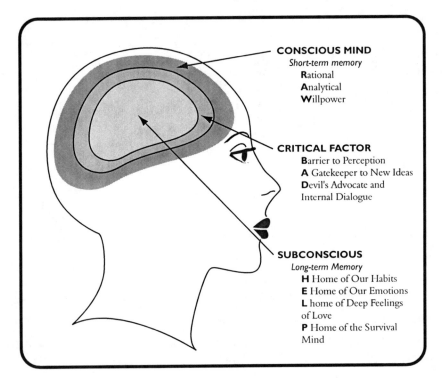

CONSCIOUS MIND
Short-term memory
Rational
Analytical
Willpower

CRITICAL FACTOR
Barrier to Perception
A Gatekeeper to New Ideas
Devil's Advocate and
Internal Dialogue

SUBCONSCIOUS
Long-term Memory
H Home of Our Habits
E Home of Our Emotions
L home of Deep Feelings
of Love
P Home of the Survival
Mind

The conscious mind is where your temporary (short-term) memory is stored. It's rational, analytical, and it also controls your willpower.

You might hear some therapists calling the critical factor the babbler, the gremlins or the chatterbox. Because it's a babbling barrier to what you perceive. It's constantly looking to disprove whatever you've heard and learned. It's forever sensing danger and reacting to fears.

The Subconscious level contains permanent memory storage, habits, emotions, and the instinct for survival. It's also responsible for the automatic functioning of your bodily systems.

The thoughts in your mind impact the operation and proper functioning of your body. Change your thoughts and you change your life.

USING YOUR MIND TO CHANGE YOUR BODY

Hypnosis can positively influence the thoughts that run through your subconscious mind. Your internal script if you will. The best way I've found to train your subconscious mind is through the daily use of self hypnosis.

Your subconscious mind controls an incredible energy force within you. Since hypnosis works by influencing your subconscious mind, it's important to gain some understanding as to what exactly the subconscious is and what it does.

The subconscious mind operates almost exactly like a computer. It has no critical or analytical ability. That only exists in the conscious mind.

The subconscious accepts any idea that you allow to enter. It isn't judging the truth or importance of it. It isn't analyzing it. If an idea gets through the Critical Factor then the subconscious automatically accepts it in the way it's been presented, for better or worse, whether it's in your best interest or not.

The subconscious will allow *any* idea to enter as long as it first passes through the Critical Factor. It doesn't matter if the thoughts are positive, negative or neutral. As computer programmers say, "Garbage in -- garbage out." If you put in garbage code, your computer will spit out garbage results.

Essentially your negative thoughts, (and that includes the negative things people have said to you as well as the negative things you have said to yourself), are what could be labeled as garbage thoughts, or "Stinkin' Thinkin" (ala Zig Ziglar.) All of those emotionally charged negative thoughts flow from your conscious mind into your subconscious and pass right through the Critical Factor.

Your subconscious automatically accepts and stores them without judgment.

Believe it or not, these perceptions all play a role in your mental programming. And they can have a very strong impact on your weight control issue. Negative thoughts provide the fertile soil in which self destructive habits can grow.

Between Two Minds

The Critical Factor level is the buffer between the conscious mind and the subconscious mind.

It serves as the gatekeeper of the mind. It keeps our mind from becoming impregnated with ideas that don't fit into reality and truth as we perceive it. It can also hold us back from changing and accepting new ideas.

THINK THROUGH IT

If you have always thought of yourself as fat, and other people have told you that you are fat, it's going to be really difficult to force your conscious mind to change the concept that it has of your being fat.

If you try to convince yourself by saying, "OK, as of now I'm not fat" your conscious mind is just NOT going to accept it. Your conscious mind simply will not accept ideas that are radically different from the ones it has already embraced as it's truth. The subconscious, on the other hand, will always win this battle of the minds.

THE SUBCONSCIOUS SIX

1. The Subconscious Mind Works Exactly Like A Computer. The subconscious mind serves as a memory storage facility, similar to the hard drive of a computer. Whatever is inputted will be saved and whatever the subconscious mind accepts it remembers forever!

The subconscious stores everything that we see, hear, taste, smell, feel, and think throughout our entire lives. It holds thoughts that we could not possibly remember consciously.

Have you ever had a problem that you couldn't solve, no matter how hard you thought about it, and then one morning the answer simply came to you as you were waking up? This is an example of your subconscious mind at work.

Before you went to sleep, you gave your subconscious mind all the information that it needed to sort through and solve, just like a computer.

To claim your free gifts (valued at $97) send a blank email to bonus@joshuaseth.com

Even though you looked at the problem from every angle and weighed the pros and cons, attended endless office meetings on the issue, and heard other people's viewpoints on the problem, your conscious mind only saw things as they are, not as they might be.

At the same time you saturated your subconscious mind with all this information and, at night while you slept, it processed it and came up with the best solution. Your conscious mind went to sleep and your subconscious mind solved the problem. When you awoke, you had your solution, automatically.

Subconscious Reprograming

This is exactly how were going to use self hypnosis to implant the conscious suggestions found throughout this book directly into your subconscious mind to help solve your weight issue!

2. The Subconscious Controls Your Involuntary Functions. Your subconscious mind controls all the involuntary functions of your body. This includes: your circulatory system, your respiratory system, your digestive system, and your elimination processes.

Imagine what life would be like if you had to consciously decide to pump your heart, consciously think "I've got to breathe right now" or "I've got to add some extra gastric acid to break up that Big Mac I just devoured".

Imagine how laborious your life would be if you had to make a conscious effort to do all of these things moment by moment! Actually, you wouldn't be very productive in life at all.

Instead, you'd be trapped inside your body, telling yourself that you must pump your blood to flow, pump your lungs to take in air, and pump digestive fluids to process your food.

We should thank our subconscious mind for taking over these functions and freeing up 99% of our time, in order that we can live, love, laugh, and enjoy being the highly advanced beings that we are. Give thanks!

3. The Subconscious Is The Seat Of Emotion. Our emotions dwell in the subconscious along with our memories and they determine the power behind our desires.

What happens with conflicting emotions?

If you are in conflict regarding your weight, you may think "I want to be thin" (the conscious desire), "but I am fat" (already accepted by the subconscious). The subconscious "internal script" always wins over the conscious desire.

When thoughts and feelings are in conflict with each other, emotions win out over logic. Imagination wins out over willpower. And the subconscious wins out over the conscious.

The conscious application of willpower is easily conquered by the subconscious power of emotion.

4. The Subconscious Mind Controls Your Imagination. Your subconscious mind is in charge of your imagination. Don't think you have one? That's not possible. Everyone has an imagination and that imagination affects your life every single day.

Emotions reside in the subconscious and so does your imagination. When you are in an emotional state, you can be motivated to proceed in the direction of whatever you are imagining as real. Emotions are the fuel for the subconscious while imagination is the language of the brain.

The subconscious doesn't "think" in the usual way, it only reacts. It can't distinguish between reality and fantasy. It perceives all the information it recieves through the senses as real.

Your subconscious can be your greatest ally in your quest for success and self-improvement. It's always wisest to have your subconscious on your side, your emotions engaged with your goals, and your imagination manifesting it into your life. Here's a good example of your imagination at work:

Grab a 2 x 4 piece of wood (maybe 8 or 12 feet long), and lay it down on the ground.

Now walk across it.

That was pretty easy, right?

OK, now let's see how well your imagination can work on this test, with a minor variation. Imagine that you take that plank of wood and you lay it in the gap between two rooftops, 20 feet off the ground. Now walk across it!

Can't do it, can you?

Perhaps, you're afraid because you imagined that that you'd fall down 20 feet. But, you haven't fallen yet, right? This is simply your imagination working overtime on the thought of falling.

If you imagine a picture of yourself falling to the ground, it creates a fear response which can cause physical reactions despite nothing having actually occurred.

5. The Subconscious Mind Automates Habitual Behavior. All of our habitual behavior, including dressing, walking, and driving a car, is carried out by the subconscious mind.

At some point, we consciously learned these activities and had to focus on carrying them out, but soon they became habits.

Now, we do these things automatically, without ever thinking about them. Our subconscious already has those thought patterns in place. These patterns direct our lives until we replace them with new patterns.

6. The Subconscious Mind Directs Your Life. The subconscious mind directs energy towards achieving your goals based on your focused thoughts.

Thoughts and behaviors are the expression of our energy. Your subconscious mind constantly sends energy towards a goal, and unless it is told specifically what to focus on, it will choose its own point of focus or adopt the focus of someone else who's influencing your reality.

This focus, when created by someone else, can usurp your best interests and last for years. In the field of hypnosis these are called "Imprints" and result in behaviors that are the product of other people's scripts. For instance, going into a certain line of work because it was expected of you. Or eating to excess because you accepted other people's judgement of you as a fat person.

Nothing is true until we make it true. You can chose to direct your subconscious mind toward becoming the best and highest version of yourself, not the fulfillment of how other people perceive you to be. In the next chapter I will show you how to unlearn negative habits and imprints and replace them with productive, proactive behaviors. It's time to reprogram your subconscious mind to automatically achieve your weight loss goals.

CHAPTER 11
10 Simple Steps To Your Weight Loss Success

"Non Satis Scire"

That's Latin for "To know is not enough". What it means it that you must also do. These ten steps are the information you need to know. Hypnosis is the vehicle that will get you to do them consistently.

The following 10 steps comprise the foundation of the suggestions I embed in my weight loss hypnosis sessions.

While your conscious mind may initially resist these suggestions, your subconscious will accept them without judgement. So the most effective way to learn these steps is through repetition while in a hypnotic state.

A sample hypnosis script is provided for you at the end of this book. Feel free to modify it with the following 10 steps, focusing on the issues that are most relevant to you.

To claim your free gifts (valued at $97) visit www.joshuaseth.com/bonus

Step Number One

Stress Less

Stop stressing out, stop worrying – stress and worry do not do you any good whatsoever. We're not in control of most things in our lives. However, we are in control of ourselves. And we are responsible for ourselves.

The first thing you can do to help yourself lose weight is to decrease the level of stress in your life. Stress and weight gain are inextricably linked to one another.

When you feel out of control and get stressed out, you go into what's called fight or flight mode.

Human beings are hardwired to the fight/flight mode response and have been for thousands of years. Emotions trigger chemical releases that cause stress responses.

If a mountain lion is above you on a hill, and is going to jump down and attack you, you either need to fight for your life or run for your life. This is called the "fight or flight" response. It's not a decision. It's a highly adrenalized automatically produced response to stress.

Now that fight or flight reaction was a very good idea when our ancestors either had to hunt to survive or become hunted themselves. Fight or flight responses rarely make sense today. There's no one to fight and nowhere to run, but the stress that produces them is a constant byproduct of our modern way of life.

Today, we're trapped in our cars on the freeway, and we're late to work. The cell is ringing and shaking, and there's traffic all around. You're sure your boss is going to yell at you when you arrive.

To claim your free gifts (valued at $97) send a blank email to bonus@joshuaseth.com

And, you had an argument with the kids before you left. Whatever -- stress, stress, stress, stress, stress, stress, stress!

What happens with all that pressure that you've been suppressing? It just builds up inside of you? You must find a way to vent it before you blow, right?

How do you let off steam? If you don't know how to vent in a productive, proactive way, it builds up. It builds up, and you release it through comfort eating, through emotional eating typically, right?

Even if you don't do that, even if you don't release the stress by eating to change your emotional state, all that adrenaline still has to go somewhere.

You become saturated with adrenaline when you're constantly stressed. There is no place for it to go so you stuff it down into your waistline, you stuff it with snacks, cakes, candies, pies, ice cream, and more. Right? This is what happens, you either get sick or you put on weight.

You get tension headaches, your back gets thrown out of whack, and you become more susceptible to disease. There are many different physical maladies that result from being stressed out.

You feel bad and you put on weight, which makes you feel lethargic and depressed, so you eat more to feel better and the vicious cycle continues.

So Number One is to learn to stress less. Hypnosis is the best way I've ever found to systematically relax on a daily basis so you never find yourself eating as an emotional response to stress again.

To claim your free gifts (valued at $97) send a blank email to bonus@joshuaseth.com

Step Number Two

Drink Lots Of Pure Clean Water

Now don't get all caught up in the whole 8-10 glasses a day thing. What are you supposed to do, carry around a little pad of paper and mark off each time you drink a glass of water? "Okay, I'm on glass number 4 ½, right?" I've never understood that.

Just drink water! Whenever you are thirsty drink water. Avoid drinking anything else for the greatest effect because water is a body cleanser, a purifier, and a natural body detoxifier. Freshly squeezed vegetable and fruit juices are second. Green tea makes the list too, but that's about it.

Whenever you're hungry, drink water before you eat. It's important. Drink a glass of pure water ½ hour before you start eating. I'll tell you why in a moment.

But first I want you to understand how much better water is than just about anything else you can drink. Almost everything else you drink is really a diuretic. Sugary drinks, caffeinated drinks, teas, coffees, soft drinks especially, they're diuretics – they will make you pee, and that will make you more thirsty and you'll keep on drinking more sugary drinks, caffeinated drinks, teas, coffee, soft drinks.

And by the way, did you know that your body cannot tell the difference between hunger and thirst? Your mind processes both hunger and thirst pretty much the same way.

Many times when you think you're hungry you're really just dehydrated and thirsting for water. So here's a simple way to know the difference between hunger and thirst ... drink a glass of water about 20-30 minutes before you eat.

Room temperature water is best. Twenty to thirty minutes before mealtime drink a glass of water and you may find that you're really not hungry after all, you were just thirsty.

Even if you're still hungry, you'll be more satisfied with much less food because your stomach has begun to process the food you ate with the water you drank. And it's mostly water you've consumed.

So drink more water. Its a very simple tip that will help you to eat less food and feel more satisfied with what you are eating at the same time. Sound good?

Step Number Three

Eat More Frequently

Many people skip meals when attempting to lose weight. They mistakenly think that if they can just go without food for most of the day then they will naturally begin to slim down. As you now know, your body doesn't work that way. When you are hungry and you don't eat your metabolism slows down, you go into starvation mode, and it becomes harder to reach your weight loss goals.

Don't ever deny yourself food. Don't allow yourself to enter the starvation mode. I'd like to refer to something I call "skinny chick syndrome", okay?

The skinny chick is the one that most people are catty about and point at from across the room saying "look at her, look at that skinny chick, she eats whatever she wants, she eats whenever she wants, it's just not fair, it's not fair!"

To claim your free gifts (valued at $97) send a blank email to bonus@joshuaseth.com

Just step back and detach for a moment. Be nonjudgmental about this skinny chick and just observe her eating behavior. You'll probably discover that your skinny chick is a grazer.

Those who tend to be naturally skinny like that never develop hang-ups about food, so they don't deny themselves the foods they want when they're hungry. They're skinny so they don't have to. They eat when they're hungry and that's the best thing you can do too.

When you eat when you're hungry, that means you'll eat several small meals a day, 5-6 meals a day typically. Smaller meals spaced out every few hours is the best.

Doing that maintains a more balanced blood sugar level, so you're not peaking and crashing all the time. Plus, you're not going into comatose mode after lunch because you just had too much food as a result of being starved in the first place.

Remember, with several small meals a day, you never allow yourself to get that hungry in the first place, you just graze. Does that make sense?

I'm not talking about snacking between meals. I'm talking about having more meals, regularly spaced out throughout the day. More meals, smaller meals, every few hours. Don't let yourself get too hungry or too full.

Be balanced.

Step Number Four

Eat Without Guilt

You won't go hungry unless you want to. You won't starve. So you don't have to worry about that. You can eat when you're hungry, okay? It's all right.

Don't ever feel guilty about eating. And don't have hang-ups about eating any particular types of food.

If your body is craving a certain food, you might need the nutrients in it, so go ahead and eat. Now if it's chocolate or sugar, that sort of thing, that's a sweet craving and that's what the hypnosis CDs are for. One of them is devoted exclusively to that issue. Additionally, you can watch the acupressure tapping technique demonstrated in the bonus video I've created especially for readers of this book. That's one of the free gifts I'll give you when you visit www.joshuaseth.com/bonus

So cravings have the potential of being for nutrients that you need, or thay can be sweet cravings, which are usually foods that you are either addicted to or allergic to. That's a different matter, but it's very easy to get over any type of cravings by using hypnosis.

In general though, eat what your body tells you it wants and don't confuse those messages by creating a bunch of artificial food hang-ups. Get out of your head and reconnect with your body.

Step Number Five

Be Grateful & Enjoy Your Food

Be appreciative, be grateful, give thanks for what you eat and enjoy what you're eating.

You might notice that a religious person will sit down and pray before a meal. What's happening with that 'grace' is they're becoming more attuned, more present in that moment, and more thankful for the food that they're going to eat. Simultaneously, they're thankfully aware that they are not one of the more than two billion people on the planet that are going to go without for that particular meal.

When you are more grateful for the food that you're taking into your body, I believe that you actually benefit from it more.

Step Number Six:

Slow Down Your Rate Of Eating

This is the most important of all the steps because if you just do this one thing, I promise that you will lose weight.

Whenever the food is in your mouth, it does not necessarily need to be on a fork in your hand. When the food is in your mouth put the fork down.

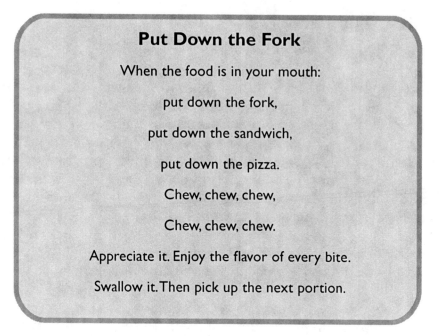

Put Down the Fork

When the food is in your mouth:

put down the fork,

put down the sandwich,

put down the pizza.

Chew, chew, chew,

Chew, chew, chew.

Appreciate it. Enjoy the flavor of every bite.

Swallow it. Then pick up the next portion.

People tend to eat as fast as they can. They have food in their mouths and as they begin chewing, they're automatically loading their fork with more food.

If you do that, you are feeding your machine without thought, without pause, without pleasure. You're not really even enjoying the flavor of the food when you do that. Slow down!

Slow down. Learn to appreciate every single bite. Become conscious and aware of each and every bite that you put in your mouth. Chew, and chew some more, and with each bite that you are conscious of you will start to lose weight. You will become more satisfied while consuming less food.

Step Number Seven

20 Minutes Of Patience

Because people used to eat more slowly, our body/mind connection between having a full stomach and realizing it with our thoughts takes about 20 minutes. It takes 1/3 of an hour to mentally realize that feeling of being "full" has traveled from your stomach to your brain. By slowing down your rate of eating, you're giving yourself a chance to become aware of when you're actually full instead of eating to excess. If you can, extend your meals by 20 minutes and eat more slowly.

Have you ever been busily eating because you felt hungry one minute and then the next minute you felt absolutely stuffed?

That's simply because you're eating too fast. Yes, your mother was right when she told you to "Slow down and chew your food!"

By the way, keep in mind that chewing foods and breaking them down with your saliva is more effective than breaking them down with your stomach acids. Therefore, the more you chew your food, the better your digestion will be as well.

Step Number Eight

Leave A Little Food On Your Plate At Every Meal

You don't ever need to eat all the food on your plate. I've eaten out at a lot of restaurants. I travel over 250 days a year. I probably eat about 700 meals in restaurants and hotels each and every year.

If you couldn't tell from my photo, I'm not a particularly big guy, but I get the same amount of food on my plate as everyone else, including those guys who are a full foot taller than me.

Now if I ate all the food that was put on my plate at restaurants, I would be just as big as everyone else, but not as tall.

I remember hearing stories of children raised in the US after World War II and how their parents told them to clean their plates because kids were starving in Europe.

Later on it was starving in Korea, Vietnam, Africa, and elsewhere. The story has no basis in your own eating habits and is only a manipulative ploy that parents use to get their children to clean their plates.

Personally, I cannot physically eat all the food on my plate *and neither can you.* The portions are way too big in this country.

In order not to eat all the food on your plate you're going to have resign your membership in The Clean Plate Club that you've been a member of since you were a little kid.

Resign your membership in The Clean Plate Club today. That starving kid in Somalia you were told about, they're never going to get the food from your plate anyway – no matter what mom or dad may have said. So, don't feel guilty about not finishing all the food on your plate. It's already been wasted, it may as well not end up on your waist.

Here's what hypnotists call reframing: Instead of thinking guilty thoughts about not finishing the food on your plate, think this instead, "Imagine how much more food there would be in the world for everyone else if we would all just eat a little bit less".

One way I suggest doing this when you're out at a restaurant with someone else, is to split the meal. Simply share the meal upfront by having the waiter serve it for two. Tell your waiter, when ordering, that you want two plates and you're going to share the meal. If you're still hungry after you finish your portion, you can always order more food.

Whenever I'm traveling alone and I'm at a restaurant, I tell the waitress to put half of the meal in a 'to go' bag right when I place the order. Requesting 50% to go reduces any temptation to eat it all at one sitting, because I've only got half of it on my plate to start with.

One other thing that you can do: whenever you eat anything, for the next 21 days at every meal that you eat, leave some food left over on your plate. A crust of bread, a leaf of lettuce, a little corner of that sandwich, just a little. Okay? This is so your eyes see that you're no longer a part of The Clean Plate Club.

Your brain will create new associations and then, over time, you'll automatically stop having those guilty thoughts.

Step Number Nine

Exercise.

I'm not talking about doing anything difficult like competing in an iron man triathlon. I'm not even talking about going to the gym every day.

But hey, if you like going to the gym, fantastic, more power to you. It's always beneficial to aerobically exercise your body and build your muscle mass. Muscle weighs more than fat though so you may not lose as much weight (but you will be healthier).

Most of us, on the other hand, don't tend to go to the gym and work out. Maybe we get the gym membership as part of our New Year's resolution, but we won't use it. According to the International Health, Racquet & Sportsclub Association, 50% of all new health club members quit within the first six months of signing up.

What I want to discuss with you is a way to move your body and increase your metabolism without having to join a gym or spend a lot of time and money. I guarantee that it will also improve your attitude, enhance your mood and reduce your weight all at the same time. And you can do all of this for less than ten bucks.

Go to any sporting goods store or corner drug store and they'll have this little thing called a pedometer.

I wear mine all the time. Actually, as of this morning, I've already done 2,358 steps so far today. It's still kind of early.

My goal is to go for 10,000 steps a day every day, and that's what I suggest you do as well. 10,000 steps a day. Most Americans tend to take 8,000 steps a day. So all I'm asking you to do is take an extra 2,000 steps a day. Two thousand steps a day, by the way, is about a mile.

Now if I ask you to walk an extra mile every day, somehow that might seem like work. Walking an extra mile a day sounds like a lot. It's not. But it sounds like it might be, right?

But if I ask you to walk an extra 2,000 steps a day, it becomes a game or a challenge. It becomes a fun activity that you can break it up throughout the day.

Take the stairs instead of the elevator. Park a little bit further away from the entrance to your home or office. Walk to the end of the hall and back.

Before you know it you've walked those 2,000 extra steps and you've completed 10,000 for the day, and guess what – it didn't stress or strain you and you feel great from doing it. No extra work at all, just a fun little challenge that you can easily accomplish.

So what I suggest you do is go out today and get yourself a pedometer. You might even want to get one for every member of your family.

You won't need a pedometer that counts calories or anything complex like that, just get one that counts steps.

- **Week #1**   Reset your pedometer, the first thing every morning, and notice how many steps you are taking throughout the day. Observe the numbers and learn your walking activity level.

- **Week #2**   Move in the direction of walking 10,000 steps daily.

- **Week #3**   Maintain 10,000 steps a day, or increase the amount according to your comfort level and continue that process.

It'll become second nature to you before you know it. And, there are all kinds of benefits that you will experience as well, like being in a great mood and feeling an increased sense of personal well being.

By going the extra mile, you're metabolizing your food better, your metabolism is increasing and that is giving you more energy.

The mere fact that you're moving your body a little bit more every day will release additional endorphins, which will make you feel happier as well.

A pedometer: it's inexpensive and will help you move your body and increase your metabolism each and every day.

To claim your free gifts (valued at $97) send a blank email to bonus@joshuaseth.com

Step Number Ten

Use Self Hypnosis Daily.

The easiest way to put the preceding steps into action is to reenforce them through the use of hypnosis on a daily basis. Remember, all hypnosis is self hypnosis. You do it to yourself. Whether by choice or by accident, the suggestions you give to your subconscious mind will determine your behaviors. In the next chapter I will give you a self hypnosis script that you can use to program all of these suggestions into your subconscious mind to achieve permanent weight loss success.

CHAPTER 12
The Self Hypnosis Solution

The daily use of self-hypnosis will keep you motivated, continuously reprogram your eating habits, eliminate emotional eating, and help you become consciously aware of what you are putting in your mouth.

You'll develop a highly positive mindset as you systemize this process for a minimum of 21 days in a row. That will reenforce the suggestions and allow them to automatically become a part of your life. A new lifestyle that you have created because ...

Above all you love yourself. You realize that you're a good person, with an enhanced self esteem simply because you've taken the responsibility to make these positive improvements in your life, and in the process you are attracting positive people and positive opportunities into your life as well. As you start to feel better about yourself, people will start to feel better about you too!

You can use the self hypnosis script provided later in this chapter as a guide for creating your own weight loss hypnosis recording. Simply read it into a tape recorder, iPod mic, or computer. You may want to mix it together with some relaxing music as well. Play it back to yourself every day for 21 days straight.

To claim your free gifts (valued at $97) visit www.joshuaseth.com/bonus

Many people prefer to use the Weight Loss Hypnosis System CDs I've created. If you don't like the sound of your own voice (a common phenomenon), have trouble making the recording yourself, or simply want to take advantage of my professionally produced 6 CD set, you can get 50% off the normal price by going to www.WeightLossHypnosisSystem.com.

Before you begin to use the weight loss hypnosis script that follows, it's important that you complete a few preliminary tasks to insure your safety and success.

FIRST: See Your Doctor

It's extremely important to verify that you are in good health by seeing your doctor first. Discuss with your physician the importance of eating properly and explore various options for exercise.

Warning: It's possible to hurt yourself if you've been without physical activity for a long period of time and you suddenly start an exercise routine without preparation or warm-ups. An ounce of prevention is worth a pound of cure!

Discuss with your physician how much weight you need to lose. Be realistic about it. The amount will differ from one person to the next. Create an achievable goal and then hit it.

You may be surprised to discover that in order to achieve a healthy physique, especially in women, you may not have to lose as much weight as you originally thought. Perhaps you only need to tone up. An extra 2,000 steps a day helps.

SECOND: Sign Your Personal Commitment Contract

If you have not already signed this contract with yourself do so now.

Don't skip this step unless you intend to waste your time and your investment in this system. This contract is vital to your successful weight loss.

Without signing this contract and making this commitment, without your desire to participate actively in the program, you will not lose weight. Not on this program or any other program in which you choose to participate. As with all self improvement endeavours, you will get out of it what you put into it. So give it your all.

It's important to understand that you can't lose the weight for someone else. This contract is signed by you and is a commitment that you are making to yourself and for yourself alone.

- If your spouse is nagging you to lose weight, don't do it for them.

- If your friends are bugging you, don't do it for them either.

- You are losing weight for yourself first and foremost

This is a contract, a commitment, an agreement between you and yourself . Leave everyone else out of it.

Committing your weight loss goals to paper via a signed contract is very important because it will drastically increase the likelihood of your achieving them.

Setting goals and writing them down is a fundamental component of success in all areas of life. Whether your personal goal weight is 120 pounds, 150 pounds or 200 pounds, you need to identify exactly what it is and write it down.

It's unwise to make your weight loss goal something like, "By the end of the week I will have dropped 10 pounds."

Your weight is going to drop at different rates of speed during the first few days than it will later on in the program.

For instance, you may lose weight at a rapid rate the first few days, especially if you have a lot of weight to lose. Then, your weight may plateau for a while.

Create realistic goals, then write them down and sign your name to them. When you've done this, rip your signed contract out of the book and post it on your refrigerator so you and everyone else in your home can see it. Hold yourself accountable. Do it now.

The Weight Loss Hypnosis Solution
PERSONAL COMMITMENT CONTRACT

I, _____, am ready to free myself of my excess

weight. I am ready to be a slimmer more healthy person!

On the date of _____ , I am taking control of my

life and my weight and will have completed my New You Weight

Loss Hypnosis pre-session work and begin participating with

my Sensory Enhanced Hypnosis Sessions.

I'm making this commitment to lose_____ pounds for myself,

my health and my future and know I will be successful.

_____   _____

Your Signature   Date

_____

Witness

Post this contract with yourself in a visible location.

To claim your free gifts (valued at $97) send a blank email to bonus@joshuaseth.com

THIRD: Select Your Weight Loss Start Date

Grab your calendar and take a look at it right now. We're going to circle you're weight loss start date on it. It's best to select a start date when you don't have much going on. Don't start when out of town guests are coming to visit, or when you're going on a vacation. Christmas and Thanksgiving probably aren't the best days to start either. Too much pressure :-)

Pick a date and stick to the contract. This is the day you will begin to transform your life. Stick with that date. Do not change it.

When that day rolls around, don't say to yourself, "Oh, I think I'll start tomorrow." You'll only be postponing your future as a slim and healthy person if you do.

Circle your start date on the calendar now.

FOURTH: Complete Your Worksheets

Let's go over each pre-session worksheet. You'll get additional copies of all these forms when you sign up at www.joshuaseth.com/bonus

Daily Food Diary

This Seven Day Food Diary must be used prior to beginning the program. It is provided so that you can write down EVERYTHING you eat and drink during the week before you begin your self hypnosis sessions.

After seven days, look at your diary. You'll probably see patterns developing, such as afternoon or evening snacking, eating when you are stressed out or upset, or grabbing "just a few" candies from the candy dish every time you pass by it at the office. It is important to write down *everything* you eat and *everything* you drink.

Everything counts. Look up the calorie count of your morning latte and your sodas and keep the numbers in mind.

Far too many people think that because they are drinking something and not actually chewing it, it has no calories. That is simply not true. Those caramel frappuccinos add up quick.

I recommend that you continue tracking your eating habits for an entire month if possible. You'll find great value in continuing to assess your eating habits over time. At the end of the month, you'll have the satisfaction of being able to look back over your diary to see how you've changed for the better.

The Weight Loss Hypnosis Solution
DAILY FOOD DIARY

Write down everything you eat in this diary. Make sure you note the amounts of the foods you are eating. You may be surprised at what you are actually consuming!

Date:_____

Breakfast: _____

_____

Mid-Morning: _____

Lunch: _____

_____

Afternoon: _____

Dinner:_____

_____

After Dinner: _____

Miscellaneous: _____

Water: _____

To claim your free gifts (valued at $97) send a blank email to bonus@joshuaseth.com

Your Personal Journal

Explore your emotional state and dig deep to see how you really feel about yourself. Introspection will help you determine if your emotions are a factor contributing to your weight issues. Write out of all the reasons why you want to be thin.

Ask yourself:

• Will being thin make me happier with myself?

• Will I be able to participate in activities I can't partake in now?

• Do I want to lose weight for health reasons?

• Do I want to lose weight for my spouse or my kids?

• Do I want to lose weight for my career?

• How will I feel about myself when I lose the weight I desire?

The Weight Loss Hypnosis Solution
Personal Thoughts Journal

Use these pages to write down your thoughts about yourself. Think about the reasons you may be afraid to lose weight, the changes your weight loss would bring, and if there are any underlying reasons why you would not want to lose the excess weight.

_____

_____

_____

_____

_____

_____

_____

_____

_____

_____

_____

To claim your free gifts (valued at $97) send a blank email to bonus@joshuaseth.com

Your Daily Action Item

You'll be creating daily goals to take action on throughout your weight loss hypnosis program. It's a good idea to give it some thought beforehand. Make small, achievable, daily goals for yourself. These goals will move you forward toward your larger target of achieving your ideal weight.

These mini-goals might be something like passing the candy jar at work without taking any or walking around the block after dinner.

Weekly Reward Journal

Use this form to plan and track your non-food rewards at the end of each time period for successfully accomplishing all of your daily action items.

These rewards can be fun little perks, like sleeping in for an extra hour on the weekend, or reading a good book, or pampering yourself with a long bubble bath.

Begin to think about things you that enjoy doing that are not food-related.

For the monthly portion of the reward sheet, the rewards can be bigger than they are on the weekly portion. Maybe your monthly reward can be buying yourself a new outfit, going to the movies (but no popcorn or snacks!), or taking an outdoor excursion. It's totally up to you.

Remember to make the goals you set for yourself realistic and easy to achieve on a daily basis.

Here Are Some Daily Goal Ideas:

1. Passing up the candy dish at work

2. Not eating any of the cookies you bake for your kids

3. Not participating in the potluck at work

4. Taking a 10 minute brisk walk after you eat lunch

5. Passing on the cream and sugar in your morning coffee

6. Eating only half the food portion on your dinner plate

7. Taking the stairs instead of the elevator

8. Walking your dog at some point during the day

9. Passing on the popcorn and snacks at the movies

10. Drinking water instead of soft drinks

List Other Ideas Here:

1.

2.

3.

Simple Goals To Start

By now you can see what types of goals are appropriate to set for yourself. They are easy, yet each goal is a stepping stone to achieving your target weight.

Set one goal for each day of the week. Everyone can accomplish ONE thing daily, right?

Look at the list above and modify it so it relates to you and your own life. Write down one goal per day and associate it with a non-food reward. One a day, no more.

The Weight Loss Hypnosis Solution
Weekly Reward Journal

Week of_____
This week's reward is_____
This month's reward is_____

Monday Action Item:_____
Today's Reward is_____
I completed my Action Item _____ I did not complete my action item _____

Tuesday Action Item:_____
Today's Reward is_____
I completed my Action Item _____ I did not complete my action item _____

Wednesday Action Item:_____
Today's Reward is_____
I completed my Action Item _____ I did not complete my action item _____

Thursday Action Item:_____
Today's Reward is_____
I completed my Action Item _____ I did not complete my action item _____

Friday Action Item:_____
Today's Reward is_____
I completed my Action Item _____ I did not complete my action item _____

Saturday Action Item:_____
Today's Reward is_____
I completed my Action Item _____ I did not complete my action item _____

Sunday Action Item:_____
Today's Reward is_____
I completed my Action Item _____ I did not complete my action item _____

To claim your free gifts (valued at $97) send a blank email to bonus@joshuaseth.com

Monthly Analysis

It's important to review your progress and celebrate your achievements on a regular basis. At the end of each month, complete this form and appreciate how far you've come. Life is a process of "becoming". Each month that you stick to your weight loss plan brings you closer into alignment with your ideal self.

The Weight Loss Hypnosis Solution
Monthly Analysis

Month:_____

Weight at the beginning of the month: _____

Amount of weight I lost this month: _____

Weight at the end of the month: _____

This month I had _____ entries in my Personal Thoughts Journal.

This month I set _____ Action Items.

This month I completed _____ Action Items.

This is how I am rewarding myself for achieving my goals this month:

This is how I feel about my success this month:

These are things I need to work on for next month:

To claim your free gifts (valued at $97) send a blank email to bonus@joshuaseth.com

> ## Do Unto Yourself
>
> When you work on your weight loss,
> your weight loss will work for you.
>
> When you go to work on your weight loss plan,
> your weight loss plan will go to work on you.
>
> Whatever good things you do for your own health,
> you do for yourself and for your loved ones.

Three Steps A Day To Melt The Weight Away

1. Fill out your Action Item and Rewards Report. Do this every day until you complete this entire program. Don't skip a day.

2. Participate once a day with your Weight Loss Hypnosis Session. Listen for at least twenty-one days straight. If you skip a day. don't get down on yourself, just get back on track and listen for another 21 days.

3. Track your progress with your Daily and Monthly Reports.

Having A Challenge?

If you are experiencing difficulty or having trouble staying focused, distract your mind with some light exercise (a brisk 10-20 minute walk can do wonders) or by reading through some informational weight loss articles. There are lots of them on my blog at www.JoshuaSeth.com

To claim your free gifts (valued at $97) send a blank email to bonus@joshuaseth.com

Your Weight Loss Success List

Before you begin the weight loss hypnosis process that follows, make sure you can put a check mark √ by each of the following:

☐ I have visited my doctor and discussed nutrition, exercise and my weight loss goals

☐ I have signed my Weight Loss Commitment Contract

☐ I have listened to the Fast Start Audio*

☐ I have listened to the Hypnotic Pre-talk Audio*

☐ I have circled my start date in the calendar

☐ I have completed the Seven Day Food Diary

☐ I have filled out my Personal Thoughts Journal

☐ I have taken time to visualize myself as thin. If I am not a visual person, I have thought about what it would sound like to hear compliments when I begin to lose weight, or what it would feel like to accomplish something I currently find difficult to do, such as walking up a flight of stairs without breathing hard, etc.

☐ I have defined my daily and weekly goals

☐ I have made a commitment to create a daily action item

☐ I have read this book from cover to cover

☐ I am excited about creating my new life!

To claim your free gifts (valued at $97) send a blank email to bonus@joshuaseth.com

Your Sample Hypnosis Script

Here is a weight loss hypnosis script that you can record in your own voice. You will notice that the hypnotic language patterns used in the following passages do not follow normal linguistic guidelines. Sentence structures are convoluted, syntaxes are mixed up, and concepts are delivered in an unusual style. It is presented this way on purpose. Hypnotic language is different from day to day language. Record it as it is written, without attempting to "fix" it, for the best results.

NOTE: I've already recorded a set of 6 weight loss hypnosis sessions that I'm making available at a 50% discount for readers of this book. If you prefer to use my version instead of making your own, please visit www.WeightLossHypnosisSystem.com.

Start Recording:

It is now time for your sensory enhanced self-hypnosis session. Let's begin. You should never participate with this program while you're driving or operating any machinery. You should now be seated or comfortably reclined.

(START RELAXATION MUSIC)

Begin by taking in a deep breath. Breathe in through your nose and let it out through your mouth. That's good.

Now take in another deep breath through your nose and this time as you let it out through your mouth, make the sound, "HA" like in Hawaii. That's right.

Take twice as long to exhale as you do to inhale and on your next breath breathing in deeply through your nose, hold it for a moment. And as you exhale through your mouth saying the HA sound simply close your eyes and let all stress just go from your body. Like water running off a duck's back all stress just flows right out of your body. That's right.

And you're now becoming totally relaxed, totally free from any concern. Totally relaxed. Very good. And as you continue breathing slowly and deeply, as you become even more relaxed now, you now want to take a moment to thank your unconscious mind, that we are talking to right now, for taking such good care of you all this time. That's right.

Just take a moment to thank your unconscious for loving you and caring for you constantly. Every moment of every hour of every day. Every minute, every second, year after year loving and caring for you as it does even now.

Every minute of every day and every night, just as it does now, your unconscious mind loves you and cares for you and assists you in doing everything. Everything it can do to allow these changes to be accepted and allow the changes to take place right now. That's right.

As we address your unconscious mind even now the changes are taking place. As you are changing, you are changing and you know it.

And now that you know these thoughts, the ones that you know -- you know. It's time for you to be aware of how these changes are affecting you right now. As you are aware of these changes now, you become aware that these changes are beginning in you and you can begin to see them. Because, even as you see the changes and you can feel the changes that you see, you feel the changes that you feel-- and as you see them you feel them, and you become aware of how great and complete these changes are, they are already becoming a part of you.

To claim your free gifts (valued at $97) visit www.joshuaseth.com/bonus

Now that you are aware of these changes that you have been making and are making, throughout these changes, right now you have changed. As you are aware of the changes now, and as you become even more aware of the depth of your breathing you realize how fully relaxed you are. Perhaps even more relaxed than the last time you were this relaxed. And even more relaxed now. And now even more. And as you are aware of how relaxed you are becoming you realize that you are so relaxed. And you realize that you no longer understand how relaxed you can become.

Because you are so relaxed and because you are becoming even more relaxed with every easy breath you take, you can allow all of the other positive, creative thoughts to manifest into your physical world.

As the positive results begin to manifest, to change, to take form, and even as they do -- you find yourself in greater control of your life mentally, emotionally and physically too.

From this point forward, you consume fewer calories than you burn. You reduce your food intake. You feel good about yourself. You are strong. You are strong. You are. You love yourself.

You know the way to natural thinness. You see yourself now, having achieved your goal weight. You control your life. The outcomes of your life are based on your decisions. From this day forward you make smart decisions and feel confident about yourself. You feel good about your life and your future. You do. You have the discipline to establish a healthy eating pattern.

Eating less, feeling more satisfied. Enjoying making healthy food chocies day by day.

Today your decision is to be committed to achieving your weight goals. You see myself succeed. You feel yourself succeed. You know in your heart that you deserve to be fit and trim and healthy. Free of the burden of weight you once had.

To claim your free gifts (valued at $97) visit www.joshuaseth.com/bonus

You control my life and your emotions. You know you have experienced the burden of extra weight all that you need too. It is now time to experience the naturally thin you, full of energy and life and living stress free.

You're gaining control.......you are in control......Your self esteem is strong.....Your stress levels are low and easily manageable.......your weight loss creates success....daily...... now........daily you find yourself drawn to activity.... you do some physical activity daily......... you feel good about yourself and don't find hunger to be an issue at all...... you burn more calories than you consume........hear it......(pause)............feel it (pause).......experience it (pause).......see it (pause)......... hear the sounds (pause).......experience....the positive (pause).....see..... you..... weighing less..........getting trim......slim........the new you (pause).

You feel so good. You enjoy life more. You are healthier. Your body feels good. You are more full of life because you have made a commitment to achieve your goals. It's wonderful to feel so good about yourself and so proud of what you can achieve, for yourself, your family, your loved ones and your future.

You find yourself eating less and being more satisfied. You find yourself eating smaller portions and liking it better. You find that you have much more energy now that you are eating less and feeling more satisfied. You always eat one bite at a time. Thinking about each bite. Feeling the texture and flavor of the food in your mouth. You never eat in front of the television. You are tired of all the unhealthy foods you used to eat. You eat smaller portions and feel so good in every way.

Every day and in every way you are getting better and better.

(END RELAXATION MUSIC)

Soon, when I count from 1-5 you will return to being fully awake and aware. You will feel very good about yourself and this weight loss hypnosis process. By the time I reach the number 5 you will be fully awake and refreshed. You will be more aware and awake than when you started this session. Your eyes will open easily only when you have accepted the belief of each suggestion you have been given.

1... more alert now wanting to move...2... feeling refreshed...3... becoming more aware of your surroundings...4... starting to yawn and blink and stretch and move and...5... wide awake, opening up your eyes and noticing how good you feel.

Welcome back! Thank you very much for allowing me to help you today and I look forward, as I'm sure you do, to participating with this program again tomorrow.

(END RECORDING)

Congratulations

I congratulate you on your decision to take control of your life and create a healthier YOU! Many people talk about losing weight but you are different. You are doing something about it.

Remember, I am here to support you. In the coming days ahead things may seem a little difficult and certain steps may seem unimportant, I can assure you that they are not. Put these self hypnosis suggestions into practice every day for 21 days straight and you will be amazed by the results.

You are heading in the right direction to achieve permanent weight loss and become the person that you truly are inside. However, you must be willing to stick with the process and participate fully. Don't give up and don't lose sight of where we are heading together. Keep the end result in mind at every step along the way.

Many people before you have successfully achieved their weight loss goals with this system and I am are certain you are joining their ranks.

Now it is time to get started. Soon you will look back on this day as a new beginning, the day you learned how to lose weight to become the new you!

I hope you will allow me to continue this relationship with you through *The Weight Loss Hypnosis 6 CD System*. There is information about this additional resource on the following pages.

I will always do my best to respect your needs, merit your trust, and value our relationship to the fullest.

I look forward to hearing about your success. Please help inspire others by posting your weight loss success story on www.joshuaseth.com/success

Here's to a healthier, happier, thinner YOU!

Joshua Seth, CHt

Special Offer Exclusively For Owners Of
"The Weight Loss Hypnosis Solution"

Attention Frustrated Dieters...

"Have You Ever Tried To Lose Weight Through Dieting Only to Gain it All Back Again? Ever Wonder Why?"

Discover The Truth About How The Diet Industry Is Trying To Make You Even FATTER!

--by Joshua Seth, CHt

Relax.

It's not you're fault. You're not alone.

Did you know that diets are ineffective about 90% of the time?

It's simply the wrong tool for the job.

When you're hungry and you don't eat you actually slow down your metabolism and end up converting potential energy to fat. Your body thinks that food has suddenly become unavailable so it tries to protect you by storing up any unused fuel as fat! For most people, dieting actually results in weight GAIN over time.

So What Does Work For Permanent Weight Loss?

Changing your *mindset* about food. Changing your *emotional relationship* with food. And changing your *conscious appreciation* of the food you're eating. And hypnosis can help you to *make these changes quickly and easily*. This isn't just positive thinking. Positive thinking is great. it's important. But it's not enough. You can't just "think yourself thin" without the proper guidance, motivation, and instruction. And that's what I'm here to give you.

To claim your free gifts (valued at $97) visit www.joshuaseth.com/bonus

Start By Imagining Yourself Already Having Achieved Your Goal Weight

My name is Joshua Seth, Certified Hypnotherapist (CHt) and Weight Loss Expert. I specialize in helping people use the power of hypnosis to reach their goals, transform their lives, and live their dreams.

Through my live seminars I've been able to help thousands of people discover that they don't have to starve themselves to lose weight. In fact, you can still eat all the foods you love while being more satisfied eating less of them :-)

Under hypnosis, when you imagine yourself as a thin person, you really *see yourself as your ideal self* staring back at you in the mirror of your mind. You will really *hear and accept my positive words of encouragement* without critiquing yourself into inaction. You will really *feel* the *successful, happy feelings* of doing something good for yourself on a daily basis to reach your weight loss goals.

In this way you will *discover yourself quickly and easily losing the excess weight* that's been dragging you down and begin to enjoy all the fun and freedom that comes from being the new, thinner you.

The New You Weight Loss Hypnosis System

I've worked with so many people now that over time I've been able to dramatically alter traditional Hypnotherapy and NLP techniques to create the fast, permanent *New You Weight Loss Hypnosis System.*

This 6 CD self hypnosis weight loss system is designed to address the real reason people have trouble losing weight with diets... mindset and motivation.

To claim your free gifts (valued at $97) visit www.joshuaseth.com/bonus

Your Weight Loss Hypnosis System Includes...

- **6 Sensory Enhanced Hypnosis CDs**

- A Fast Start Audio Introduction (so you can take action immediately)

- **An "Introduction to Hypnosis" Pre-talk (this will set the stage for the hypnosis sessions to come)**

- The Introductory "Lose Weight and Feel Great" Self Hypnosis CD

- **A "Weight Loss Mindset" Hypnosis Session (the subconscious secrets to permanent weight loss)**

- A "Weight Loss Mindset" Conscious Programming Session (daily affirmations to keep you focused)

- **An "Exercise Motivation" Hypnosis Session (this is one of the most popular CDs in the course)**

- An "Exercise Motivation" Conscious Programming Session (that you can listen to on your way to the gym!)

- **An "Eliminate Sweets" Hypnotic Session (I used this myself to overcome cravings for chocolate)**

- An "Eliminate Sweets" Conscious Programming Session (use this before you go out to eat)

- **A "Healthy Eating Habits" Hypnosis Session (reenforces key points on a subconscious level)**

- A "Healthy Eating Habits" Conscious Programming Session

To claim your free gifts (valued at $97) visit www.joshuaseth.com/bonus

I've packaged all of the content in my *New You Weight Loss Hypnosis System* so that **for less than the cost of just one live session with a hypnotherapist, you'll receive the complete sixteen week program!** And it's guaranteed too. How many weight loss programs come with a guarantee? Not too many!

Just 20 Minutes a Day to a New "Thinner" You

It only takes about 20 minutes a day, listening to these CDs while you rest. If you cannot do that, then I'm sorry to say that this program cannot not help you. I know that time is a precious commodity, but for achieving your weight loss goals and improving your life and your health, you must be willing to participate with this program. Schedule it in the morning, afternoon or evening or fluctuate the time to fit your schedule. It's worth it. You're worth it!

Warning!

Many people start to lose weight immediately, but most people will not see any results for 2 to 3 weeks. *The New You Weight Loss Hypnosis System* is highly effective, but it is not a miracle pill. Do not expect miracles in a week. I don't offer miracles - only a real, tested, proven system.

It takes time for your body to adjust. Many people will start to lose weight from day one while others will need three weeks before the weight starts to drop. Remember, it took time for your body to get in the condition it is today, and it will take some time to restore it to normal. Through *The New You Weight Loss Hypnosis System* I will help you get there, like a good friend, supporting you every step of the way. This system works!!! Just give it a chance. YOU WILL LOSE THE WEIGHT YOU DESIRE – I guarantee it.

To claim your free gifts (valued at $97) visit www.joshuaseth.com/bonus

Your Risk Free Moneyback Guarantee to Achieve Your Weight Loss Goals

I have personally seen this program work for so many people and am so sure it will work for you too that I'm willing to go out on a limb here and take all the risk so you don't have to. First, for a full 90 days experience the weight loss and prove to yourself that this system is right for you. Enjoy all the new activities you can now participate in, all the new relationships you can have, and the wonderful way you look in your new clothes. If you then find that this system is not for you, please send it back for a full refund. I only want you to keep this system after you have proven it's value for YOU!

You already have all the information you need, contained within the pages of this book. Now put them into action with this 6 CD set. Get *The New You Weight Loss Hypnosis System* today and change your life!

You'll receive all the prerecorded hypnosis sessions you need to achieve your weight loss goals at a fraction of what you'd pay for live hypnosis sessions.

21 Days is all it takes to start making permanent changes in your weight and in your life. Today is day #1. You've read this book and made a great start. You're already on your way.

Now's the time to reenforce what you've learned with my 6 CD subconscious reprogramming system. And I'm going to make it easy for you to make this investment in your future with a special offer exclusively for the owners of this book...

To claim your free gifts (valued at $97) visit www.joshuaseth.com/bonus

Limited Time Offer

For a limited time I'm slashing $100 off the price as a special bonus to you because you've already made an investment in this book.

In the past, I've only made this special offer available to my seminar attendees. If you promise to share your weight loss success story at www.joshuaseth.com/success I'll knock a hundred bucks off the $197 list price making it just $97.

You have everything to gain and nothing to lose *but the weight.*

Remember, I'm taking all the risk and your *New You Weight Loss Hypnosis System* is 100% guaranteed.

It is my hope that this book is just the beginning of a relationship between us that will help to improve your life in many ways. I look forward to hearing of your weight loss success.

Thank you for allowing me to help you reach your goals, transform your life, and live your dreams.

Here's to a happier, healthier more successful you!

Sincerely,

Joshua Seth, CHt
www.WeightLossHypnosisSystem.com

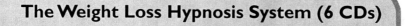

The Weight Loss Hypnosis System (6 CDs)

Special Offer for Owners of This Book: $97
Get Your Copy At This Special Reduced Rate At

www.WeightLossHypnosisSystem.com

About The Author
Joshua Seth, CHt

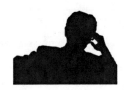

Joshua Seth is, according to TV Japan, *"The #1 American Hypnotist"*.

Joshua has toured around the world with his shows and seminars. He's the only hypnotist to have had his own prime-time TV special in Japan, not once but twice.

A partial list of his accomplishments follow:

• Joshua started Kent State University at the Age of 8.

• He later completed a 4 year degree program at New York University in only 2 years, with a double major, and graduated with honors.

• After graduation, Joshua decided he wanted to move to Hollywood and voice cartoons. It was his dream at the time, so he flew out and did it. With zero connections in Hollywood, he landed an agent within one week and soon become one of the busiest voice actors in the industry. Within a few short years he voiced the starring role of "Tai" on the #1 Saturday morning cartoon "Digimon", the starring role of "Tetuso" in the Anime classic Akira, and voiced over 50 other TV Shows and Movies (finally retiring from the field after voicing a role in the Spongebob Squarepants Movie in 2004).

To claim your free gifts (valued at $97) visit www.joshuaseth.com/bonus

- While living in LA he turned a childhood passion for magic into a six figure a year secondary career and won First Place at the Academy of Magical Arts' prestigious "Magic Castle Olympics" with his unique brand of mentalism (waking hypnosis).

- Now in his 30s, Joshua decided to leave the Hollywood scene behind and "retire" to Santa Barbara , CA. After 6 months of "retirement" (sitting on the beach every day and reading) he decided his new dream was to travel the world with his hypnosis shows and seminars and concentrate on helping other people live their dreams as has.

- Since 2005 Joshua has toured the world nonstop, headlining and consistently selling out the largest cruise-ship showrooms, corporate events, and colleges with his motivational shows and seminars. Over 200,000 people have now seen Joshua live and millions more have experienced him through his television specials.

- In 2006 Joshua starred in his own 2 hour prime-time TV Special in Japan. He returned to Tokyo to film another prime-time Network Special the following year. Both specials finished #1 in the ratings during their sweeps week premiers.

Today Joshua lectures extensively at corporations, universities, and public events on the use of self hypnosis for health and wellness, accelerated learning and sales motivation. He is the author of over a dozen personal development audio programs available at www.JoshuaSeth.com

Joshua Seth is a Master Neuro Linguistic Practitioner (NLP) and Certified Hypnotherapist (CHt) with the National Guild of Hypnotists. He is committed to helping people reach their goals, transform their lives, and live their dreams by tapping into the power of their own subconscious minds.

This is his first book.

To request Joshua for a speaking engagement for your organization, email info@joshuaseth.com

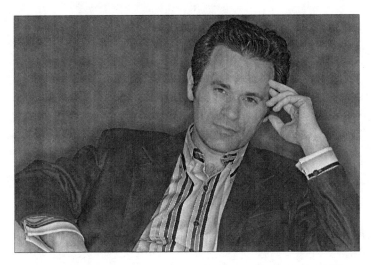

Hypnotist and Weight Loss Expert Joshua Seth, CHt

To claim your free gifts (valued at $97) visit www.joshuaseth.com/bonus

Printed in the United States
140798LV00003B/10/P